Renal Diet

90 Excellent Recipes for Stopping Kidney Disease

Table of Contents

4

Introduction

Going through life with major organ failure is a tough endeavor. You can neither do the same things nor eat the same food you used to, and if you decide to slack off from caution, it could result in an adverse outcome. Everything should be checked and done with care. To maintain a steady monitored life, you need all the information you can get from what foods to eat, what to avoid, and why certain foods need to be avoided. In a state of compromised health, the last thing you need to do is to worry aimlessly about every single aspect.

Details of certain kidney diseases are provided. All the aspects you need to know about renal dieting are provided later on, from foods to eat to how to live a much more fulfilling and stress-free life following them. Here, details of making easy to-go meals and meal planning are discussed. Also, nutritional information is given and tips on how to customize them according to your taste.

If you have been recently diagnosed with chronic kidney disease or have any illness regarding the renal system, then you first need to understand that there are thousands of people in the world living good lives with diseases such as yourself. It is not the end of the world, and with proper care and lifestyle changes, you can start living a happy life as well.

Whether recently diagnosed or not, this dieting plan will reduce the load on your kidneys and help you live a healthier life. To care for yourself is to care for your loved ones too. Your life is important to everyone that is precious to you, and you must improve as much as possible.

If making such changes seems difficult to you, then you can always ask for help from a loved one. You don't need to face all the challenges on your own, and this e-book is here to guide you through most of the aspects of the renal diet, but always ask for help or visit a doctor when you are in doubt about your health.

Chicken in Herb Sauce

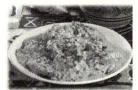

Preparation Time: 10 minutes/Cooking Time: 32 minutes/Servings – 2

Ingredients

- 2 skinless chicken breasts
- ½ teaspoon garlic powder
- ¼ teaspoon celery salt
- ¼ teaspoon ground black pepper
- ½ teaspoon paprika
- ¼ teaspoon celery seeds
- ½ teaspoon mustard powder
- 3 tablespoons lemon juice
- 2 tablespoons butter, unsalted
- 1 tablespoon parmesan cheese, grated

Asparagus and Cauliflower Tortilla

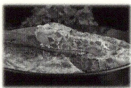

Preparation Time: 10 minutes/Cooking Time: 25 minutes/Servings – 4 pieces

Ingredients

- 2 cups asparagus, chopped and trimmed
- 1 ½ cups white onion, chopped
- 2 cups cauliflower florets, chopped
- ½ teaspoon minced garlic
- ¼ teaspoon ground nutmeg
- ½ teaspoon ground black pepper
- ¾ teaspoon salt
- ¾ teaspoon dried thyme leaves

Vegetable Paella

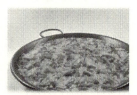

Preparation Time: 5minutes/Cooking Time: minutes/Servings – 8

Ingredients

- 4 cups cooked white rice
- 2 cups asparagus
- ½ cup white onion, chopped
- 1 cup green bell pepper, chopped
- 3 cups broccoli florets
- 1 ½ cup zucchini, chopped
- ½ teaspoon salt
- 1 tablespoon olive oil
- ½ teaspoon saffron

Mixed Berry and Fruit Salad

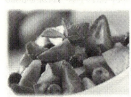

Preparation Time: 1 hour and 5 minutes/Cooking Time: 0 minutes/Servings – 4

Ingredients

- 2 cups fresh strawberries, quartered
- 10 leaves of fresh basil
- 1 cup fresh blueberries
- 1 tablespoon Splenda granulated sugar
- 2 tablespoons white balsamic vinegar
- ¼ cup almond and coconut milk blend

Blueberry Smoothie

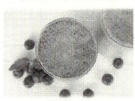

Preparation Time: 5 minutes/Cooking Time: 0 minutes/Servings – 4

Ingredients

- 1 cup frozen blueberries
- 6 tablespoons protein powder
- 8 packets of Splenda
- 14 ounces of apple juice, unsweetened
- 8 cubes of ice

Lemon and Berry Bread

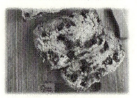

Preparation Time: 10 minutes/Cooking Time: 54 minutes/Servings – 10 slices

Ingredients

- 1 cup blueberries, fresh
- 1 ½ cups and 1 tablespoon all-purpose white flour
- 1 teaspoon baking powder
- 1 cup Splenda granulated sugar
- 1/3 cup canola oil
- 2 tablespoons lemon rind, grated
- 2 tablespoons lemon extract, unsweetened
- ½ cup lemon juice
- 4 egg whites

Renal Diet

A renal diet means to eat with an emphasis on promoting the kidney's health. It is recommended for anyone who is suffering from renal disease to reduce the progression and complications of that disease, such as electrolyte imbalance, anemia, heart disease, etc. It includes restrictions on certain micronutrients such as sodium, potassium, phosphorus, proteins, and input of fluids. A person may need to limit their consumption of vegetables, fruits, grains, and red meat. There is great importance given to what type of protein should be eaten.

Different people experience different types of renal diseases, and according to their condition, they'll need to change their diet. Some people only limit salt in their diet, and some people need to focus more on their potassium intake. You may need to discuss this with a doctor or a qualified dietitian so you can get the best possible outcome from the diet.

Micronutrients for Renal Diet

There are many nutrients that a person suffering from renal disease must monitor. Some of them are:

Sodium

Sodium is a very important micronutrient required by the body for various types of functions ranging from:

➢ Regulating fluid volume
➢ Regulating electrolytes
➢ Regulating blood pressure
➢ Regulating nerve impulses

A person going through renal disease must distance themselves from eating too much salt, as it contains high levels of sodium. Sodium causes much damage if the kidneys cannot flush out excess amounts of it. Complications may include severe swelling of the lower leg and other parts of the body, heart disease, and hypertension. It also increases thirst, which will increase the fluid load on the damaged kidney.

You can decrease your salt intake by:

➢ Decreasing your intake of processed foods since they have larger amounts of salt
➢ Eating fresh meat and vegetables with no preservatives
➢ Reading the labels on packaging for salt content
➢ Reducing salt intake to 140 mg

Potassium

This is also a very important nutrient needed for the function of the heart. It is found in many foods. It is also important for the healthy function of muscles as well. Potassium increases when kidneys do not function properly, and when this happens, it is called hyperkalemia. This can cause a series of heart problems such as:

- ➤ Arrhythmias
- ➤ Muscle degeneration
- ➤ Cardiac attack
- ➤ Paralysis

You can decrease your potassium intake by:

- ➤ Reading packaging labels for potassium levels
- ➤ Eating fresh vegetables and fruits
- ➤ Avoiding foods with a high level of potassium
- ➤ Keeping track of how much potassium you are eating in a day

Phosphorus

This is also an important micronutrient for the body's healthy functions. It is important for bone development, growth of certain organs, and connective tissues. If the kidneys are not working properly, then phosphorus will accumulate inside the body. Phosphorus takes out the calcium from the bones into the blood, making the bones weaker and increasing the level of calcium in the blood dangerously.

To keep track of phosphorus you can:

- ➤ Read the packaging labels for levels of PHOS
- ➤ Avoid eating foods with a high level of phosphorus
- ➤ Eat high quality and low-fat meat
- ➤ Eat fresh fruits and vegetables

Proteins

High levels of protein and amino acids in the blood occur when the kidneys cannot filter the excess protein properly out of the body. The broken-down proteins and their waste products circulate the body's system, causing a lot of problems. It damages the structures of the kidneys as well.

The amount of protein a person needs to consume is tricky because it depends upon the individual's condition. Overall, there is an emphasis on eating high-quality protein and reducing the amount of red meat. For complete guidance, consult a doctor or dietitian.

Water Intake

Because the kidneys are not functioning properly, excess water inside the body cannot be filtered out without the help of dialysis in extreme cases. To reduce the load on the kidneys, drink as low amounts of fluid as possible. Excess fluid can cause damage to other organs, such as the heart and lungs, by putting more pressure on them.

You can keep track of your fluid intake by:

➢ Avoiding salty and spicy foods
➢ Taking medicine with sips of water
➢ Keeping a record of fluid intake along with your food in a journal
➢ Avoiding salty condiments, such as soy sauce
➢ Drinking cold fluids
➢ Following instructions from professionals on what to drink and what not to drink

Foods for Renal Diet

Foods that you eat daily need to be regularly monitored. To encourage overall wellness, you need to take in less sodium, potassium, and phosphorus. Also, you need to eat more high-quality protein and lower your fluid uptake. Here is a detailed list of foods to eat and to avoid, which will make it easier for you to choose your next meal.

High in Sodium Foods That You Need to Avoid

➤ Different meats and sausages: chicken, pork, and cuts that have been preserved, smoked, or cured
➤ Fishes and seafood that are preserved
➤ Frozen dinners or packed dinners
➤ Canned food items like pasta or soup
➤ Salted nuts
➤ Salted and canned beans
➤ Buttermilk
➤ Cheese, cheese products, processed cottage cheese
➤ Quick bread and bread with extra salt
➤ Salted rolls
➤ Biscuits and pancakes made by self-rising flour or their mixes
➤ Salted crackers
➤ The dough of pasta, potatoes, and rice that is processed and packaged
➤ Vegetables and vegetable juices in cans

- Salted regular pickles as well as olives and other pickled vegetables
- Vegetables made with pork products
- The dough of hash browns and scalloped potatoes, which are processed and packaged
- Quick pasta meals
- Processed ketchup
- Processed and salted mustard
- Processed salsa
- Dehydrated or regular soups in cans
- Processed or regular broths
- Cup noodles processed and salted ramen mixes
- Soy sauce
- Seasoning salts
- Marinades that are salted
- Salad dressings in bottles, processed or regular
- Salad dressings with bacon
- Salted butter and margarine
- Instant custard or pudding
- Ready-to-eat cakes

Low in Sodium Foods That Should Be Taken Instead

- ➢ Fresh and frozen portions of lamb, poultry, beef, fish, shrimp, pork
- ➢ Fish and poultry, water and oil-packed, and drained; canned fish labeled as low sodium
- ➢ Eggs/egg substitutes
- ➢ Dried peas and not canned beans
- ➢ Low sodium peanut butter, almond, rice, or coconut milk, plant-based yogurts
- ➢ Low sodium cream cheese and low sodium cheeses like parmesan and ricotta
- ➢ Ready-to-eat cereals
- ➢ Rolls and bread that are not salted
- ➢ Almond, coconut, whole-wheat, low sodium plain and all-purpose white flour; low sodium corn and tortillas
- ➢ Low sodium breadsticks, crackers, unsalted popcorn, and chips
- ➢ Pasta and rice cooked without salt and low sodium noodles
- ➢ Frozen or fresh vegetables, low sodium canned vegetables without seasoning or sauce
- ➢ Low sodium vegetable juices, V-8, and low sodium tomato juice
- ➢ Low sodium pickles

- ➢ Fresh potatoes or unsalted and unseasoned frozen french fries and mashed potatoes
- ➢ Fresh and frozen canned fruits, dried fruits
- ➢ Low sodium salsa
- ➢ Low sodium soups that are canned
- ➢ Homemade broths made without any salt, and fresh ingredients
- ➢ Homemade pasta without any salt
- ➢ Low sodium soy sauce
- ➢ Low sodium seasoning and marinades
- ➢ Low sodium salad dressings
- ➢ Low sodium mayonnaise
- ➢ Unsalted butter and margarine, vegetable oils
- ➢ Homemade ketchup that is unsalted
- ➢ Unsalted mustard

High in Potassium Foods That You Need to Avoid

- ➢ Cooked spinach, artichokes, okra, broccoli, beets, fried onions, and sweet potato
- ➢ Bananas, avocados, honeydew, mango, orange, pomegranate, prune, pumpkin, coconut, and cantaloupe
- ➢ Buttermilk and shakes
- ➢ Beans, either baked or refried
- ➢ Legumes, like lentils
- ➢ Nuts, like walnuts and raisins
- ➢ Granola

- ➤ Whole grains and bran
- ➤ Fast foods, like french fries and other salty foods
- ➤ Processed meats
- ➤ Vegetable juices
- ➤ Processed sauces, like tomato sauce
- ➤ Fruit juices such as pomegranate juice, prune juice
- ➤ Creamed soups
- ➤ Yogurt, frozen and regular
- ➤ Ice creams
- ➤ Chocolate sweet dishes

Low in Potassium Foods That You Need to Eat Instead

- ➤ Asparagus, kale, broccoli, cucumber, zucchini, carrots, cabbage, bell pepper, eggplant, garlic, and lettuce
- ➤ Apples, grapes, pineapple, peaches, plum, all berries, watermelon
- ➤ Rice milk
- ➤ Greens beans and snow peas
- ➤ White rice and bread that is not whole
- ➤ Dried cranberries
- ➤ Unsalted popcorn
- ➤ Hash browns and mashed potatoes made up of leached potatoes
- ➤ Low sodium tomato and V-8 juice
- ➤ Unsalted sauces and apple sauce
- ➤ Unsalted noodles and pasta

- ➢ Non-dairy creams
- ➢ Sherbet
- ➢ Lemon and vanilla flavors instead of chocolate

High in Phosphorus Foods That Need to Be Avoided

- ➢ Some Vegetables
- ➢ Some Fruits
- ➢ Parts of chicken and other poultry
- ➢ Ham and other pork products
- ➢ Hunted animals
- ➢ Some Seafood
- ➢ Plain Bread
- ➢ Tortillas
- ➢ Muffins
- ➢ Some pasta
- ➢ Some types of rice
- ➢ Certain cheeses
- ➢ Milk
- ➢ Yogurt
- ➢ Ice cream
- ➢ Eggs
- ➢ Snacks

Low in Phosphorus Foods That Should Be Eaten Instead

- ➢ Celery, radishes, and baby carrots

- Apples, cherries, peaches, pineapples, blueberries, and strawberries
- Pot roast beef, sirloin steak
- Skinless chicken and turkey, breast and thighs
- Porkchop, mostly lean pork patty and pork roast
- Veal chop
- Wild salmon, mahi-mahi, king crab, lobster, snow crab, oyster shrimp, water, or oil-packed canned tuna
- Plain bread without salt, Italian bread, blueberry bread, sourdough bread, white bread, flatbread, wheat bread, pita bread, and cinnamon bread
- Flour tortillas, corn tortillas
- English muffins
- Macron, egg and rice noodles, spaghetti
- Couscous, long-grain white rice
- Cottage, blue, feta, parmesan, and cream cheese
- Almond, soy, and rice milk
- Non-dairy creamer
- Sorbet
- Pasteurized egg whites
- Unsalted popcorn

Kidney-Friendly Protein Options Which Are Included in the Overall Diet

- ➤ Lean beef and turkey
- ➤ Meat substitutes, like tofu and veggie sausage
- ➤ Skinless chicken breast and thigh
- ➤ Salman, trout, mackerel fish, and shrimp
- ➤ Pork chops
- ➤ Cottage cheese
- ➤ Pasteurized eggs
- ➤ Greek yogurt
- ➤ Shakes made with rice, almond, coconut, or soy milk

Kidney-Friendly Fluid Options Which Are Included in This Diet

- ➤ Fruits like apples, cherries, grapes, berries, peaches, plums
- ➤ Vegetables such as zucchini, cucumber, broccoli, cauliflower, cabbage, bell peppers, carrots, celery, lettuce, and eggplant
- ➤ Tea and coffee
- ➤ Gelatin
- ➤ Ice cubes
- ➤ Fruit juices
- ➤ Popsicles
- ➤ Milk substitutes
- ➤ Sherbet
- ➤ Low sodium soups

Awesome and Simple Renal Diet Recipes Breakfast

Apple and Cinnamon French Toast Strata

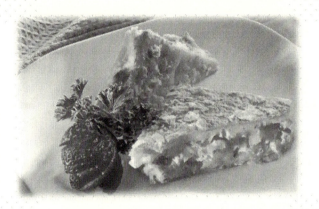

Preparation Time: 2 hours and 20 minutes/Cooking Time: 50 minutes/Servings – 12

Ingredients

- ❖ 1 ½ medium apples peeled, cored, diced
- ❖ 1 pound cinnamon and raisin loaf, diced
- ❖ 1 teaspoon ground cinnamon
- ❖ ¼ cup pancake syrup
- ❖ 6 tablespoons unsalted butter, melted
- ❖ 1 ¼ cup half-and-half creamer
- ❖ 8 ounces cream cheese, softened and cubed
- ❖ 8 large eggs
- ❖ 1 ¼ cup almond milk, unsweetened

Instructions

1. Take a 9 by 13 inches baking dish, grease it with oil, then arrange half of the bread cubes on the bottom and scatter cream cheese evenly on the top.
2. Top cream cheese with the apple, sprinkle with cinnamon, and then top with remaining bread cubes.
3. Crack eggs in a large bowl, add pancake syrup, butter, milk, and creamer, whisk until combined, pour this mixture evenly in the prepared casserole, cover it with plastic wrap, and then keep the casserole dish in the refrigerator for 2 hours.
4. When ready to cook, switch on the oven, then set it to 325°F, and let it preheat.
5. Then uncover casserole, bake for 50 minutes and when done, let it cool for 10 minutes and cut it into twelve 3 by 3-inch squares.
6. Drizzle with more pancake syrup and then serve.

Nutrition Information Per Serving

Calories – 324

Fat – 20 g

Protein – 9 g

Carbohydrates – 27 g

Fiber – 1.8 g

Cholesterol – 170 mg

Net Carbs – 25.2 g

Sodium – 280 mg

Potassium – 224 mg

Phosphorus – 224 mg

Apple and Onion Omelet

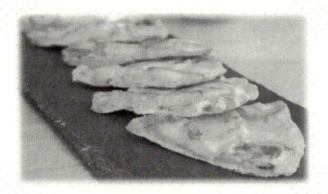

Preparation Time: 10 minutes/Cooking Time: 20

minutes/Servings – 2

Ingredients

- ❖ 1 large apple peeled, cored, sliced
- ❖ ¾ cup sweet onion, sliced
- ❖ 1 tablespoon unsalted butter
- ❖ 1/8 teaspoon ground black pepper
- ❖ 1 tablespoon water
- ❖ ¼ cup milk, low-fat
- ❖ 2 tablespoons shredded cheddar cheese, low-fat
- ❖ 3 eggs

Instructions

1. Switch on the oven, then set it to 400°F and let it preheat.

2. Crack eggs in a bowl, add black pepper and water, and whisk until beaten.

3. Take a small heatproof skillet pan, place it over medium heat, add butter and when it melts, add onions and apple and cook for 6 minutes until sauted.

4. Spread onion-apple mixture evenly, pour egg mixture over it, spread evenly, and cook for 2 minutes until eggs begin to set.

5. Then sprinkle cheese on top of eggs, transfer skillet pan into the heated oven, and bake for 12 minutes or until omelet has set.

6. When done, remove the pan from the oven, cut the omelet in half, distribute it between two plates, and then serve.

Nutrition Information Per Serving

Calories – 282

Fat – 16 g

Protein – 13 g

Carbohydrates – 22 g

Fiber – 3.5 g

Cholesterol – 303 ml

Net Carbs – 18.5 g

Sodium – 169 mg

Potassium – 341 mg

Phosphorus – 238 mg

Asparagus and Cauliflower Tortilla

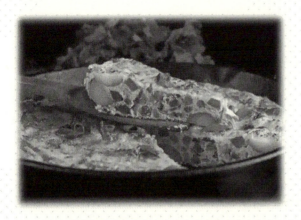

Preparation Time: 10 minutes/Cooking Time: 25 minutes/Servings – 4 pieces

Ingredients

- ❖ 2 cups asparagus, chopped and trimmed
- ❖ 1 ½ cups white onion, chopped
- ❖ 2 cups cauliflower florets, chopped
- ❖ ½ teaspoon minced garlic
- ❖ ¼ teaspoon ground nutmeg
- ❖ ½ teaspoon ground black pepper
- ❖ ¼ teaspoon salt
- ❖ ¼ teaspoon dried thyme leaves
- ❖ 2 tablespoons parsley, chopped
- ❖ 2 teaspoons olive oil
- ❖ 1 cup liquid egg substitute, low-cholesterol

- ❖ 1 tablespoon water

Instructions

1. Take a heatproof bowl, add cauliflower florets and asparagus, drizzle with water, cover the bowl with plastic wrap, pierce some holes in it and microwave for 5 minutes, or until tender-crisp.

2. Meanwhile, take a medium-sized skillet pan, place it over medium heat, add oil and when hot, add onion, and cook for 7 minutes until golden-brown.

3. Stir in garlic, cook for 1 minute until fragrant, switch heat to medium-low level, add steamed cauliflower-asparagus mixture in the pan, sprinkle with nutmeg, black pepper, salt, thyme, and parsley, and pour in egg substitute.

4. Continue cooking for 10 to 15 minutes, or until the tortilla has set and the bottom is nicely browned, and when done, slide tortilla onto a dish by running the knife along the edges.

5. Cut tortilla into four pieces and then serve.

Nutrition Information Per Serving

Calories – 102
Fat – 3 g
Protein – 9 g
Carbohydrates – 9 g

Cholesterol – 0 ml
Net Carbs – 5.2 g
Sodium – 248 mg
Potassium – 472 mg

Fiber – 3.8 g *Phosphorus – 97 mg*

Avocado Toast with Egg

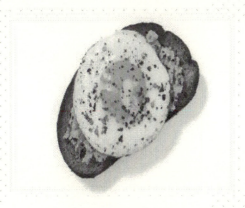

Preparation Time: 10 minutes/Cooking Time: 5 minutes/Servings – 2 toasts

Ingredients

- ❖ ½ of a medium avocado, pitted and sliced
- ❖ 1 tablespoon parsley, chopped
- ❖ ¼ teaspoon ground black pepper
- ❖ 1/8 teaspoon salt
- ❖ 1 tablespoon lime juice
- ❖ 2 tablespoons feta cheese, crumbled
- ❖ 2 eggs
- ❖ 2 slices of whole-grain bread, toasted

Instructions

1. Transfer avocado flesh to a medium bowl, mash with a fork, and then stir in salt and lime juice.

2. Spread the avocado mixture evenly onto each piece of toast, then take a skillet pan, spray it with oil and when hot, crack eggs into it and cook to the desired level.

3. Distribute eggs onto the toast, top each piece of toast with ½ tablespoon parsley, 1 tablespoon cheese, and 1/8 teaspoon ground black pepper.

4. Serve straight away.

Nutrition Information Per Serving

Calories – 225

Fat – 13 g

Protein – 12 g

Carbohydrates – 15 g

Fiber – 4.3 g

Cholesterol – 194 ml

Net Carbs – 11.7 g

Sodium – 404 mg

Potassium – 311 mg

Phosphorus – 209 mg

Baked Egg Cups

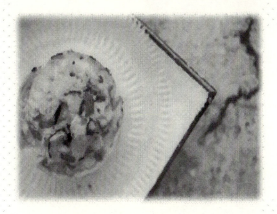

Preparation Time: 20 minutes/Cooking Time: 35 minutes/Servings – 12 muffins

Ingredients

- ❖ 1/3 cup mushrooms, diced
- ❖ ¼ teaspoon ground black pepper
- ❖ 1/3 cup green bell pepper, diced
- ❖ 1/3 cup white onion, diced
- ❖ 6 slices bacon, low-sodium
- ❖ 12 eggs

Instructions

1. Switch on the oven, then set it to 350°F and let it preheat.

2. Meanwhile, take a twelve-cup muffin tray, line it with muffin liners, and set aside until required.

3. Take a medium-sized skillet pan, place it over medium heat and when hot, add bacon slices and cook for 7 to 10 minutes, or until crispy.

4. When the bacon has cooked, transfer it to a cutting board, let it cool for 5 minutes, chop the bacon, and then transfer it to a bowl.

5. Add all the vegetables in the bowl containing bacon, stir until well mixed, and then distribute the mixture evenly between prepared muffin cups.

6. Take another bowl, crack eggs in it, add black pepper, whisk until combined, pour this mixture evenly into muffin cups, and bake into the heated oven for 25 minutes, or until firm and when the tops are golden-brown.

7. When done, let muffins cool for 5 minutes, then take them out, let the muffins cool for an additional 10 minutes, and serve.

Nutrition Information Per Serving

Calories – 80

Fat – 5 g

Protein – 7 g

Carbohydrates – 1 g

Fiber – 0.1 g

Cholesterol – 212 ml

Net Carbs – 0.9 g

Sodium – 78 mg

Potassium – 92 mg

Phosphorus – 101 mg

Breakfast Burrito

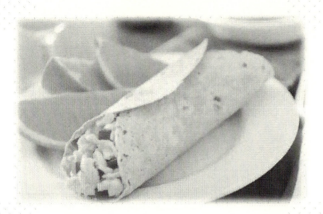

Preparation Time: 10 minutes/Cooking Time: 3 minutes/Servings – 2 burritos

Ingredients

- ❖ 3 tablespoons green chiles, diced
- ❖ ½ teaspoon hot pepper sauce
- ❖ ¼ teaspoon ground cumin
- ❖ 4 eggs
- ❖ 2 flour tortillas, burrito size

Instructions

1. Take a medium-sized skillet pan, place it over medium heat, grease it with oil, and let it get hot.

2. Crack eggs in a bowl, add chilies, hot sauce, and cumin, whisk until combined, then pour the egg mixture in the hot skillet and cook for 2 minutes, or until eggs have been cooked to the desired level.

3. Meanwhile, heat the tortillas by microwaving them for 20 seconds until hot.

4. When eggs have cooked, distribute evenly between hot tortillas and roll it up like a burrito.

5. Serve straight away.

Nutrition Information Per Serving

Calories – 366

Fat – 18 g

Protein – 18 g

Carbohydrates – 33 g

Fiber – 2.5 g

Cholesterol – 372 ml

Net Carbs – 30.5 g

Sodium – 594 mg

Potassium – 245 mg

Phosphorus – 300 mg

Chorizo and Egg Tortilla

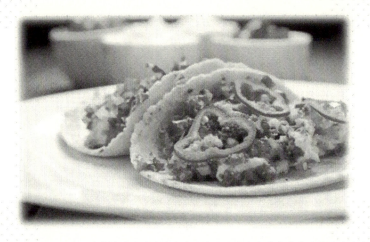

Preparation Time: 10 minutes/Cooking Time: 13 minutes/Servings – 1 tortilla

Ingredients

- ❖ 1 flour tortilla, about 6-inches
- ❖ 1/3 cup chorizo meat, chopped
- ❖ 1 egg

Instructions

1. Take a medium-sized skillet pan, place it over medium heat and when hot, add chorizo and cook for 5 to 8 minutes until done.

2. When the meat has cooked, drain the excess fat, whisk an egg, pour it into the pan, stir until combined, and cook for 3 minutes, or until eggs have cooked.

3. Spoon egg onto the tortilla and then serve.

Nutrition Information Per Serving

Calories – 223

Fat – 11 g

Protein – 16 g

Carbohydrates – 15 g

Fiber – 1.5 g

Cholesterol – 211 ml

Net Carbs – 13.5 g

Sodium – 317 mg

Potassium – 284 mg

Phosphorus – 232 mg

Cottage Cheese Pancakes

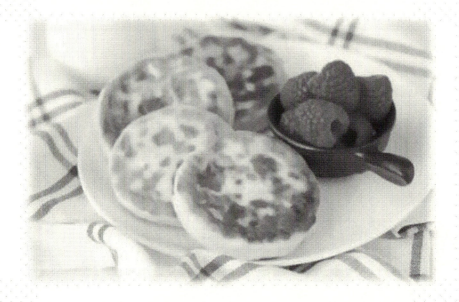

Preparation Time: 10 minutes/Cooking Time: 50 minutes/Servings – 6 pancakes

Ingredients

- ❖ 3 cups fresh raspberries, sliced
- ❖ ½ cup all-purpose white flour
- ❖ 1 cup cottage cheese, softened
- ❖ 6 tablespoons unsalted butter, melted
- ❖ 4 eggs, beaten

Instructions

1. Crack eggs in a medium-sized bowl, add flour, cheese, and butter in it, and whisk until combined.

2. Take a medium-high frying pan, grease it with oil and when hot, pour in prepared batter, ¼ cup of batter per pancake, spread the batter into a 4-inch pancake, and cook for 3 minutes per side until browned.

3. When done, transfer pancakes onto a plate, cook more pancakes in the same manner, and, when done, serve each pancake with ½ sliced raspberries.

Nutrition Information Per Serving

Calories – 253

Fat – 17 g

Protein – 11 g

Carbohydrates – 21 g

Fiber – 2 g

Cholesterol – 182 ml

Net Carbs – 19 g

Sodium – 172 mg

Potassium – 217 mg

Phosphorus – 159 mg

Egg in a Hole

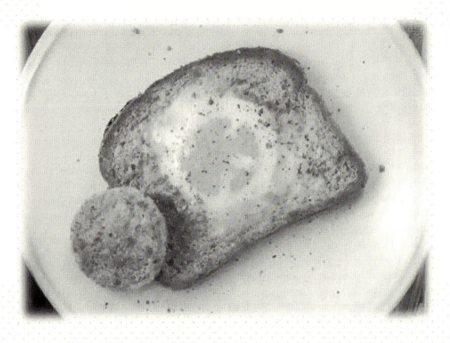

Preparation Time: 5 minutes/Cooking Time: 5 minutes/Servings – 1 slice

Ingredients

- ❖ 1 slice of white bread
- ❖ ¼ teaspoon lemon pepper seasoning, salt-free
- ❖ 1 egg
- ❖ 1 teaspoon Parmesan cheese, grated

Instructions

1. Prepare the bread by making a hole in the middle: use a cookie cutter for cutting out the center.

2. Brush the slice with oil on both sides, then take a medium-sized skillet pan, place it over medium heat and when hot, add bread slice in it, crack the egg in the center of the slice, and sprinkle with lemon pepper seasoning.

3. Cook the egg for 2 minutes, then carefully flip it along with the slice and continue cooking for an additional 2 minutes.

4. Sprinkle cheese on the egg, let it melt, then slide the egg onto a plate; serve straight away.

Nutrition Information Per Serving

Calories – 159

Fat – 7 g

Protein – 9 g

Carbohydrates – 15 g

Fiber – 0.8 g

Cholesterol – 213 ml

Net Carbs – 14.2 g

Sodium – 266 mg

Potassium – 122 mg

Phosphorus – 137 mg

German Pancakes

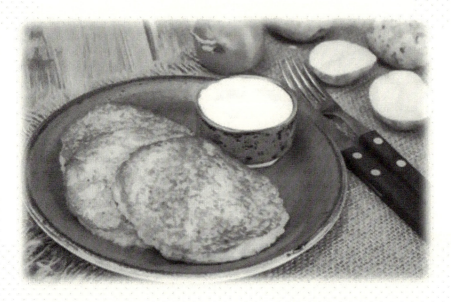

Preparation Time: 10 minutes/Cooking Time: 15 minutes/Servings – 10 pancakes

Ingredients

- ❖ 2/3 cup all-purpose flour
- ❖ ¼ teaspoon vanilla extract, unsweetened
- ❖ 2 tablespoons white sugar
- ❖ 1 cup milk, low-fat
- ❖ 4 eggs
- ❖ 1 ¼ cup cream cheese, softened
- ❖ 1/3 cup fruit jam for serving, sugar-free

Instructions

1. Prepare the batter by taking a medium-sized bowl, add flour in it along with sugar, stir until mixed, whisk in eggs until blended, and then whisk in vanilla and milk until smooth.

2. Take a skillet pan, about 8 inches, spray it with oil and when hot, add 3 tablespoons of the prepared batter, tilt the pan to spread the batter evenly, and cook for 45 seconds, or until the bottom is browned.

3. Flip the pancake, continue cooking for 45 seconds until the other side is browned, and when done, transfer pancake to a plate.

4. Cook nine more pancakes in the same manner and, when done, spread 2 tablespoons of cream cheese on one side of the pancake, fold it, and then serve with 1 tablespoon of fruit jam.

Nutrition Information Per Serving

Calories – 74

Fat – 2 g

Protein – 4 g

Carbohydrates – 10 g

Fiber – 0.2 g

Cholesterol – 76 ml

Net Carbs – 0.8 g

Sodium – 39 mg

Potassium – 73 mg

Phosphorus – 76 mg

Mushroom and Red Pepper Omelet

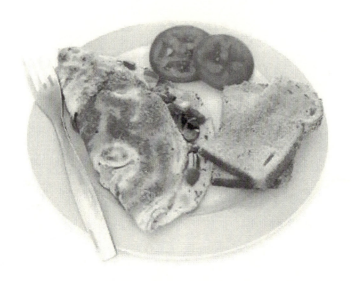

Preparation Time: 5 minutes/Cooking Time: 12 minutes/Servings – 2 plates

Ingredients

- ❖ 2 tablespoons white onion, diced
- ❖ ¼ cup sweet red peppers, diced
- ❖ ½ cup mushrooms, diced
- ❖ ¼ teaspoon ground black pepper
- ❖ 1 teaspoon Worcestershire sauce
- ❖ 2 teaspoons unsalted butter
- ❖ 3 eggs
- ❖ 2 tablespoons whipped cream cheese

Instructions

1. Take a medium-sized skillet pan, place it over medium heat, add 1 teaspoon butter and when it melts, add onions and mushrooms and cook for 5 minutes, or until onions are tender.

2. Stir in red pepper, then transfer vegetables to a plate and set aside until needed.

3. Crack the eggs in a bowl, add Worcestershire sauce, and whisk until combined.

4. Return skillet pan over medium heat, add remaining butter and when it melts, pour in the egg mixture, and cook for 2 minutes, or until omelet is partially cooked.

5. Then top cooked vegetables on one side of the omelet, top with cream cheese, and continue cooking until omelet is cooked completely.

6. When done, remove the pan from the heat, cover the filling of the omelet by folding the other half of the omelet, sprinkle it with black pepper, and then divide omelet into two.

7. Serve straight away.

Nutrition Information Per Serving

Calories – 199

Fat – 15 g

Protein – 11 g

Carbohydrates – 4 g

Fiber – 0.6 g

Cholesterol – 341 ml

Net Carbs – 3.4 g

Sodium – 276 mg

Potassium – 228 mg

Phosphorus – 167 mg

Apple and Zucchini Bread

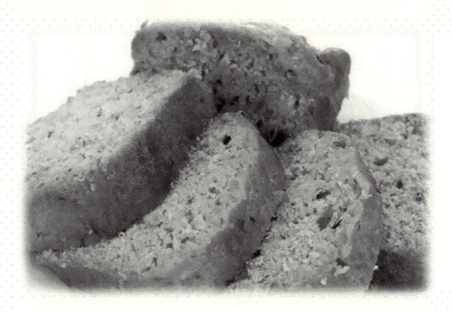

Preparation Time: 15 minutes/Cooking Time: 50 minutes/Servings – 36 slices

Ingredients

Loaves

- ❖ 2 cups zucchini, grated
- ❖ 3 ½ cups and 2 tablespoons all-purpose white flour
- ❖ 1 cup apples, chopped
- ❖ 1 ½ teaspoons baking soda
- ❖ ¾ cup white sugar
- ❖ ½ teaspoon salt
- ❖ 3 teaspoons ground cinnamon

- ❖ ¾ cup Splenda brown sugar blend
- ❖ 1 teaspoon vanilla extract, unsweetened
- ❖ ½ cup olive oil
- ❖ 4 eggs

Topping
- ❖ ¼ cup all-purpose white flour
- ❖ 2 tablespoons unsalted butter, cold
- ❖ ¼ cup brown sugar

Instructions

1. Switch on the oven, then set it to 350°F and let it preheat.
2. Meanwhile, take two 9-by-5 inches loaf pans, spray them with oil, sprinkle with 2 tablespoons of flour, and set aside until needed.
3. Crack eggs in a large bowl, add vanilla, eggs, oil, white sugar, and ¾ cup brown sugar, and whisk until combined.
4. Take another large bowl, add remaining flour in it, stir in baking soda, 2 tablespoons cinnamon and salt until mixed, and then gradually stir the flour mixture into egg mixture until incorporated. Don't over-mix.
5. Then fold in grated zucchini and chopped apples until mixed, distribute the batter evenly between the two prepared loaf pans and bake in the heated oven for 40 minutes.

6. Meanwhile, prepare the topping by placing all of its ingredients in a food processor and pulse for 1 to 2 minutes, or until the mixture resembles crumbs.

7. After 40 minutes of baking, top the loaves evenly with the topping and continue baking for 10 minutes, or until the top has turned golden-brown, and loaves passed the skewer test (if the skewer comes out clean from the center of the bread).

8. When done, let the loaves cool in the pan for 10 minutes, then take them out from the pan and cool them for 20 minutes on the wire rack.

9. Cut each loaf into eighteen slices, each about ½-inch thick, and then serve.

Nutrition Information Per Serving

Calories – 134

Fat – 5 g

Protein – 2 g

Carbohydrates – 20 g

Fiber – 0.6 g

Cholesterol – 25 ml

Net Carbs – 1.4 g

Sodium – 93 mg

Potassium – 53 mg

Phosphorus – 28 mg

Spicy Corn Bread

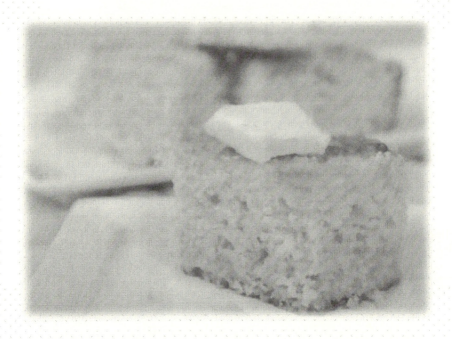

Preparation Time: 15 minutes/Cooking Time: 30 minutes/Servings – 8 pieces

Ingredients

- ½ cup scallions, chopped
- ¼ teaspoon minced garlic
- ¼ cup carrots, grated
- 1 cup cornmeal
- 1 cup all-purpose white flour
- 2 teaspoons baking powder
- ¼ teaspoon ground black pepper
- 1 tablespoon white sugar

- ❖ 1 teaspoon red chili powder
- ❖ 1 egg
- ❖ 2 tablespoons canola oil
- ❖ 1 egg white
- ❖ 1 cup of rice milk

Instructions

1. Switch on the oven, then set it to 400°F and let it preheat.

2. Meanwhile, take a large bowl, add cornmeal and flour in it, and then stir in black pepper, red chili powder, baking powder, and sugar until combined.

3. Take another large bowl, add egg and egg white in it, whisk in oil and milk until blended, and then gradually whisk this mixture into the flour mixture until incorporated.

4. Add carrots, scallions, and garlic, stir until just mixed, then take an 8-inch baking pan, grease it with oil, pour the prepared batter in it, and bake for 30 minutes until bread is firm and the top has turned golden-brown.

5. When done, let the bread cool for 10 minutes in the pan, then take it out, cut the bread into eight pieces, each about 2-by-4 inches, and serve.

Nutrition Information Per Serving

Calories – 188

Fat – 5 g

Protein – 5 g

Carbohydrates – 31 g

Fiber – 2 g

Cholesterol – 26 ml

Net Carbs – 29 g

Sodium – 155 mg

Potassium – 100 mg

Phosphorus – 81 mg

Pumpkin Bread

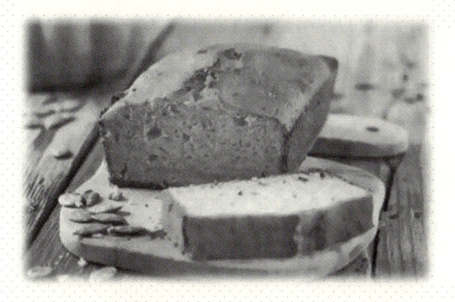

Preparation Time: 20 minutes/Cooking Time: 45 minutes/Servings – 30 slices

Ingredients

- ❖ 3 ½ cups all-purpose white flour
- ❖ 2 cups pumpkin
- ❖ 1 teaspoon ginger powder
- ❖ ½ teaspoon baking powder
- ❖ 2 teaspoons baking soda
- ❖ 1 teaspoon cinnamon
- ❖ 1 teaspoon salt
- ❖ 2 cups white sugar

- ❖ ½ cup olive oil
- ❖ 2/3 cup water
- ❖ 4 eggs

Instructions

1. Switch on the oven, then set it to 350°F, and let it preheat.

2. Meanwhile, take a large bowl, crack eggs in it, add pumpkin, sugar, oil, and water and whisk until beaten.

3. Gradually beat in flour, baking soda, ginger, cinnamon, and salt until smooth, distribute the batter evenly between three loaf pans and then bake for 45 minutes until the top has turn golden-brown and loaves pass the skewer test (if the skewer comes out clean from the center of the bread).

4. When done, let the loaves cool in the pan for 10 minutes, then take them out from the pan and cool them for 20 minutes on the wire rack.

5. Cut each loaf into ten slices and then serve.

Nutrition Information Per Serving

Calories – 145

Fat – 5 g

Protein – 3 g

Carbohydrates – 24 g

Fiber – 0.8 g

Cholesterol – 28 ml

Net Carbs – 23.2 g

Sodium – 171 mg

Potassium – 61 mg

Phosphorus – 38 mg

Sour Cream and Apple Bread

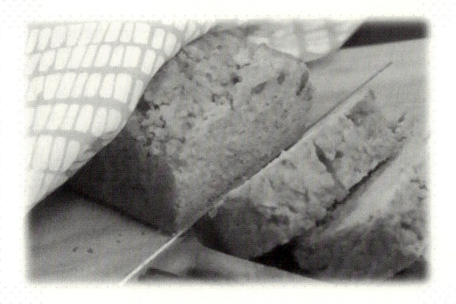

Preparation Time: 20 minutes/Cooking Time: 55 minutes/Servings – 10 slices

Ingredients

- ❖ 1 cup diced apple
- ❖ 1 2/3 cups all-purpose white flour
- ❖ ¼ teaspoon salt
- ❖ ¾ teaspoon baking powder
- ❖ ½ cup white sugar
- ❖ ¼ teaspoon baking soda
- ❖ ½ teaspoon ground cinnamon
- ❖ ¼ cup canola oil
- ❖ 2 egg whites

- ❖ 1/3 cup applesauce, unsweetened
- ❖ ½ cup confectioners' sugar
- ❖ 2/3 cup sour cream, reduced-fat
- ❖ 6 tablespoons water

Instructions

1. Switch on the oven, then set it to 350°F and let it preheat.
2. Meanwhile, take a large bowl, add flour in it and then stir in baking soda and powder, salt, and cinnamon until mixed.
3. Take a separate bowl, add oil in it, beat in sugar until well combined, then gradually beat in flour mixture, egg whites, and applesauce until incorporated and fold in apples and sour cream until just mixed.
4. Take an 8.5-by-4.75 inches loaf pan, grease it with oil, pour the batter in it and then bake for 55 minutes until the top has turned golden-brown and loaf passes the skewer test (if the skewer comes out clean from the center of the bread).
5. When done, let the loaf cool in the pan for 10 minutes, then take it out from the pan and cool them for 20 minutes on the wire rack.
6. Cut the loaf into ten slices and then serve.

Nutrition Information Per Serving

Calories – 135   *Cholesterol – 6 ml*

Fat – 3 g

Protein – 3 g

Carbohydrates – 24 g

Fiber – 1 g

Net Carbs – 23 g

Sodium – 139 mg

Potassium – 74 mg

Phosphorus – 48 mg

Strawberry Bread

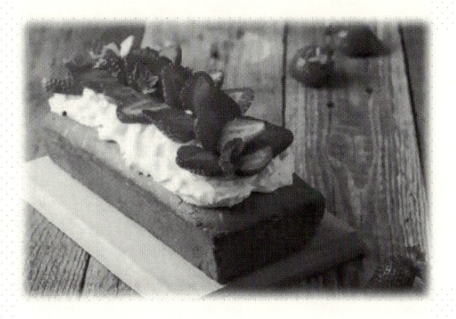

Preparation Time: 10 minutes/Cooking Time: 50 minutes/Servings – 20 slices

Ingredients

- ❖ 3 cups all-purpose white flour
- ❖ ¾ teaspoon salt
- ❖ 1 teaspoon baking soda
- ❖ ¼ teaspoon ground cinnamon
- ❖ 2 cups white sugar
- ❖ 1 cup canola oil
- ❖ 4 eggs
- ❖ 2 ½ cups fresh strawberries, chopped

Instructions

1. Switch on the oven, then set it to 350°F and let it preheat.

2. Crack eggs in a medium bowl, beat in oil until incorporated, and then stir in berries until mixed.

3. Take a separate large bowl, add flour in it along with remaining ingredients, stir until mixed, then make a well in the center, pour in egg batter and mix well until blended. Don't over-mix.

4. Take two 9-by-5 inches loaf pans, distribute the batter evenly between them and then bake for 60 minutes until the top has turned golden-brown and loaves pass the skewer test (if the skewer comes out clean from the center of the bread).

5. When done, let the loaves cool in the pan for 15 minutes, then take them out from the pan and cool them for an additional 20 minutes on the wire rack.

6. Cut each loaf into ten slices and then serve.

Nutrition Information Per Serving

Calories – 254

Fat – 12 g

Protein – 3 g

Carbohydrates – 33 g

Fiber – 0.8 g

Cholesterol – 42 ml

Net Carbs – 32.2 g

Sodium – 157 mg

Potassium – 64 mg

Phosphorus – 39 mg

Zucchini Bread

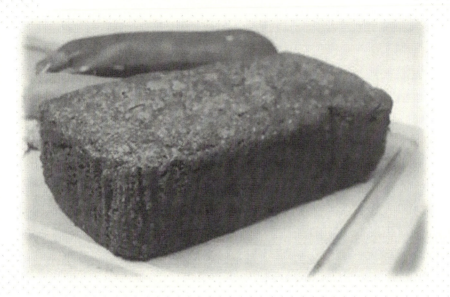

Preparation Time: 20 minutes/Cooking Time: 60 minutes/Servings – 24 slices

Ingredients

- ❖ 2 cups zucchini, grated
- ❖ 3 cups all-purpose white flour
- ❖ 1 teaspoon salt
- ❖ 1 ½ teaspoons baking soda
- ❖ ¾ cup Splenda granulated sweetener
- ❖ 1 ½ teaspoons pumpkin pie spice
- ❖ 2 tablespoons lemon juice
- ❖ 1 teaspoon vanilla extract, unsweetened
- ❖ ¾ cup honey

- ❖ 1/3 cup olive oil
- ❖ 4 eggs
- ❖ 1/3 cup applesauce, unsweetened

Instructions

1. Switch on the oven, then set it to 325°F and let it preheat.
2. Meanwhile, take a large bowl, add flour in it and then stir in salt, Splenda, baking soda, and pumpkin pie soda until mixed.
3. Take a separate bowl, crack eggs in it, beat until blended, stir in remaining ingredients until incorporated and then stir this mixture gradually into flour mixture until combined. Don't over-mix.
4. Take two 8.5-by-4.5 inches loaf pans, distribute the batter evenly between them and then bake for 60 minutes until the top has turned golden-brown and loaves pass the skewer test (if the skewer comes out clean from the center of the bread).
5. When done, let the loaves cool in the pan for 10 minutes, then take them out from the pan and cool them for an additional 20 minutes on the wire rack.
6. Cut each loaf into twelve slices and then serve.

Nutrition Information Per Serving

Calories – 156

Fat – 4 g

Protein – 3 g

Carbohydrates – 27 g

Fiber – 0.6 g

Cholesterol – 35 ml

Net Carbs – 26.4 g

Sodium – 160 mg

Potassium – 70 mg

Phosphorus – 38 mg

Lemon and Berry Bread

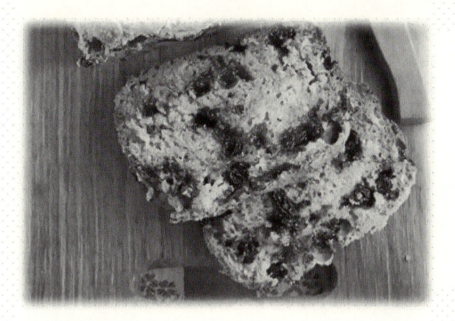

Preparation Time: 10 minutes/*Cooking Time:* 54 minutes/*Servings* – 10 slices

Ingredients

- ❖ 1 cup blueberries, fresh
- ❖ 1 ½ cups and 1 tablespoon all-purpose white flour
- ❖ 1 teaspoon baking powder
- ❖ 1 cup Splenda granulated sugar
- ❖ 1/3 cup canola oil
- ❖ 2 tablespoons lemon rind, grated
- ❖ 2 tablespoons lemon extract, unsweetened
- ❖ ½ cup lemon juice
- ❖ 4 egg whites

❖ ½ cup milk, low-fat

Instructions

1. Switch on the oven, then set it to 350°F and let it preheat.

2. Meanwhile, take a large bowl, add 1 ½ cups flour in it and then stir in the baking powder until mixed.

3. Take another bowl, add oil in it and beat in egg white, lemon extract, and 2/3 cup Splenda until well combined.

4. Then whisk in flour mixture alternating with milk until just mixed (do not over-mix), and fold in lemon rind and berries until combined.

5. Take a 9-by-5-3 inches loaf pan, grease it with oil sprinkle with 1 tablespoon flour, pour in prepared batter in it, and bake for 50 minutes until the top has turndc golden-brown and loaf passes the skewer test (if the skewer comes out clean from the center of the bread).

6. Meanwhile, prepare the glaze by taking a saucepan, place it over medium heat, add remaining Splenda in it, then stir in lemon juice and cook for 4 minutes, or until the sugar has dissolved.

7. When the bread has baked, let the loaf cool in the pan for 10 minutes, then take out the bread, poke holes into the top, at the 1-inch interval, and pour prepared glaze on the bread.

8. Cut the loaf into ten slices and then serve.

Nutrition Information Per Serving

Calories – 229

Fat – 8 g

Protein – 3 g

Carbohydrates – 36 g

Fiber – 0.8 g

Cholesterol – 0 ml

Net Carbs – 35.2 g

Sodium – 78 mg

Potassium – 89 mg

Phosphorus – 41 mg

Apple Muffins

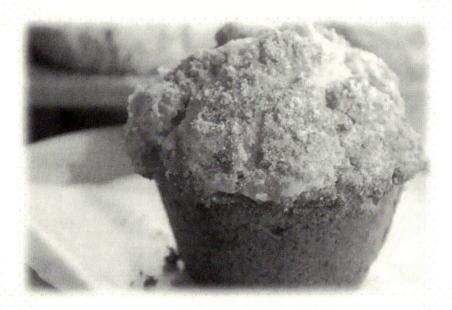

Preparation Time: 15 minutes/Cooking Time: 20 minutes/Servings – 12 muffins

Ingredients

- ❖ 1 ½ cups all-purpose white flour
- ❖ 1 ½ cups diced apple
- ❖ 1 teaspoon baking soda
- ❖ 1 cup and 1 teaspoon Splenda granulated sugar
- ❖ 1 ½ teaspoons cinnamon
- ❖ 1 tablespoon vanilla extract, unsweetened
- ❖ ½ cup canola oil

- ❖ ¼ cup water
- ❖ 2 eggs

Instructions

1. Switch on the oven, then set it to 400°F and let it preheat.

2. Meanwhile, take a large bowl, crack eggs in it and then beat in oil, 1 cup sugar, water, and vanilla until mixed.

3. Take a separate bowl, place flour in it, stir in 1 teaspoon cinnamon, and baking soda until mixed, then gradually stir this mixture into the egg mixture until combined and fold in apples.

4. Take a twelve-cup muffin tray, line the cups with a muffin liner, and distribute prepared batter into the cups.

5. Stir together remaining sugar and cinnamon, sprinkle this mixture on top of muffins and then bake for 20 minutes until the top has turned golden-brown, and muffins pass the skewer test (if the skewer comes out clean from the center of muffins).

6. When done, let muffins cool in the tray for 10 minutes, then take them out and serve.

Nutrition Information Per Serving

Calories – 162

Fat – 10 g

Protein – 3 g

Carbohydrates – 15 g

Fiber – 0.8 g

Cholesterol – 35 ml

Net Carbs – 14.2 g

Sodium – 117 mg

Potassium – 46 mg

Phosphorus – 34 mg

Gingerbread Muffins

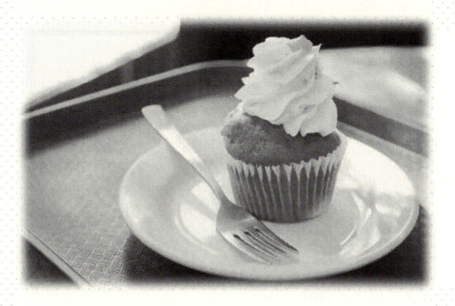

Preparation Time: 15 minutes/Cooking Time: 20 minutes/Servings – 12 muffins

Ingredients

- ❖ 2 cups all-purpose white flour
- ❖ 4 teaspoons ginger powder
- ❖ 1 ½ teaspoons ground cinnamon
- ❖ 1 tablespoon baking powder
- ❖ ½ cup brown sugar
- ❖ 6 tablespoons canola oil
- ❖ 4 tablespoons corn syrup

- ❖ 2 eggs
- ❖ ¾ cup milk, low-fat

Instructions

1. Switch on the oven, then set it to 400°F and let it preheat.

2. Meanwhile, take a medium-sized bowl, crack eggs in it and then beat in oil, sugar, corn syrup, and milk until combined.

3. Take a separate large bowl, place flour in it, stir in cinnamon, baking powder, and ginger until mixed, make a well in the center, pour in the egg mixture and whisk until incorporated. Don't over-mix.

4. Take a twelve-cup muffin tray, line the cups with a muffin liner, distribute prepared batter into the cups and then bake for 20 minutes until the top has turned golden-brown and muffins pass the skewer test (if the skewer comes out clean from the center of muffins).

5. When done, let muffins cool in the tray for 10 minutes, then take them out and serve.

Nutrition Information Per Serving

Calories – 216

Fat – 8 g

Protein – 4 g

Carbohydrates – 32 g

Fiber – 0.8 g

Cholesterol – 32 ml

Net Carbs – 31.2 g

Sodium – 154 mg

Potassium – 80 mg

Phosphorus – 81 mg

Banana and Chocolate Chip Muffins

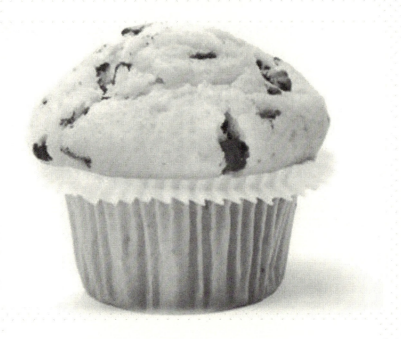

Preparation Time: 10 minutes/Cooking Time: 15 minutes/Servings – 12 muffins

Ingredients

- ❖ 2 large bananas, peeled and mashed
- ❖ ½ cup chocolate chips, semi-sweet
- ❖ 2 tablespoons honey
- ❖ ½ teaspoon baking soda
- ❖ ½ teaspoon ground cinnamon
- ❖ 1 teaspoon vanilla extract, unsweetened
- ❖ 1 cup peanut butter
- ❖ 2 eggs

Instructions

1. Switch on the oven, then set it to 400°F and let it preheat.
2. Meanwhile, take a large bowl, place bananas in it, mash with a fork, then add remaining ingredients (except for chocolate chips), whisk until incorporated, and then fold in chocolate chips until just mixed.
3. Take a twelve-cup muffin tray, line the cups with a muffin liner, distribute prepared batter into the cups and then bake for 15 minutes until the top has turned golden-brown and muffins pass the skewer test (if the skewer comes out clean from the center of muffins).
4. When done, let muffins cool in the tray for 10 minutes, then take them out and serve.

Nutrition Information Per Serving

Calories – 222

Fat – 14 g

Protein – 6 g

Carbohydrates – 18 g

Fiber – 2 g

Cholesterol – 100 ml

Net Carbs – 10160 g

Sodium – 167 mg

Potassium – 247 mg

Phosphorus – 102 mg

Blueberry Dream Muffins

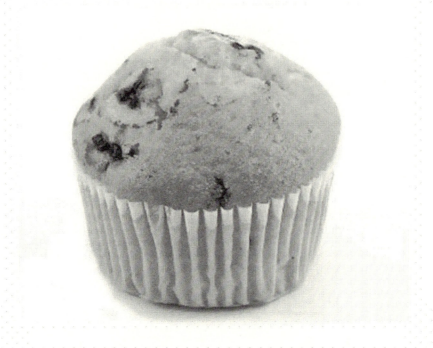

Preparation Time: 10 minutes/Cooking Time: 25 minutes/Servings – 12 muffins

Ingredients

- ❖ 1 cup frozen blueberries
- ❖ 2 cups all-purpose white flour
- ❖ ½ cup Splenda granulated sugar
- ❖ 2 teaspoons baking powder
- ❖ 1 tablespoon lemon zest
- ❖ 1 egg, beaten

- ❖ ¼ cup olive oil
- ❖ 1 cup of rice beverage

Instructions

1. Switch on the oven, then set it to 375°F and let it preheat.

2. Meanwhile, take a large bowl, add flour in it, and stir in sugar and baking powder until mixed.

3. Take a separate medium-sized bowl, crack the egg in it, whisk in lemon zest, oil and rice beverage until combined, then whisk this mixture into flour mixture until incorporated and fold in berries until mixed.

4. Take a twelve-cup muffin tray, line the cups with a muffin liner, distribute prepared batter into the cups and then bake for 25 minutes until the top has turned golden-brown and muffins pass the skewer test (if the skewer comes out clean from the center of muffins).

5. When done, let muffins cool in the tray for 10 minutes, then take them out and serve.

Nutrition Information Per Serving

Calories – 171

Fat – 5 g

Protein – 3 g

Carbohydrates – 28 g

Fiber – 1 g

Cholesterol – 18 ml

Net Carbs – 27 g

Sodium – 95 mg

Potassium – 39 mg

Phosphorus – 53 mg

Cranberry Muffins

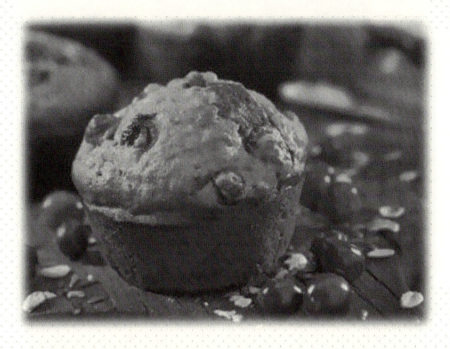

Preparation Time: 15 minutes/Cooking Time: 20 minutes/Servings – 12 muffins

Ingredients

- ❖ 1 cup fresh cranberries, chopped
- ❖ 1 ¾ cups all-purpose white flour
- ❖ 7 tablespoons Splenda granulated sugar
- ❖ ¼ teaspoon salt
- ❖ 2 teaspoons baking powder
- ❖ ¼ cup olive oil
- ❖ ¾ cup cranapple juice
- ❖ 1 egg, beaten

Topping

- ❖ 3 tablespoons all-purpose white flour
- ❖ 2 tablespoons unsalted butter
- ❖ ¼ teaspoon ground cinnamon
- ❖ 3 tablespoons brown sugar

Instructions

1. Switch on the oven, then set it to 400°F and let it preheat.

2. Meanwhile, prepare the topping and for this, take a small bowl, place flour in it, stir in cinnamon and sugar until mixed, and then cut the butter in it until mixture resembles crumbs.

3. Prepare the muffins by taking a large bowl, add flour in it, and then stir in Splenda, baking powder, and salt until mixed.

4. Take a separate bowl, crack eggs in it, whisk in oil and cranapple juice until blended, then pour this mixture into the flour mixture until incorporated and fold in cranberries until just mixed.

5. Take a twelve-cup muffin tray, line the cups with a muffin liner, distribute prepared batter into the cups, sprinkle with topping, and then bake for 20 minutes until the top has turned golden-brown and muffins pass the skewer test (if the skewer comes out clean from the center of muffins).

6. When done, let muffins cool in the tray for 10 minutes, then take them out and serve.

Nutrition Information Per Serving

Calories – 187

Fat – 7 g

Protein – 3 g

Carbohydrates – 29 g

Fiber – 1 g

Cholesterol – 19 ml

Net Carbs – 28 g

Sodium – 134 mg

Potassium – 45 mg

Phosphorus – 48 mg

Pumpkin Muffins

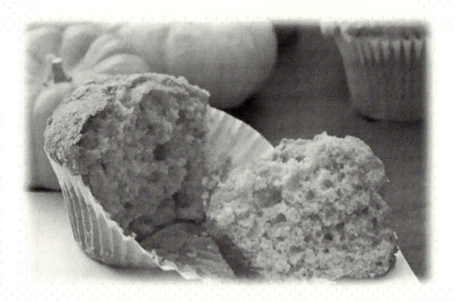

Preparation Time: 10 minutes/Cooking Time: 18 minutes/Servings – 12 muffins

Ingredients

- ❖ ½ cup pumpkin
- ❖ 1 tablespoon pumpkin pie spice
- ❖ ½ teaspoons baking soda
- ❖ 1/3 cup chocolate chips, semi-sweet
- ❖ 1/3 cup maple syrup
- ❖ 1 cup peanut butter

Instructions

1. Switch on the oven, then set it to 400°F and let it preheat.

2. Meanwhile, take a large bowl, add all the ingredients in it except for chocolate chips, whisk until incorporated, and then fold in chocolate chips until just mixed.

3. Take a twelve-cup muffin tray, line the cups with a muffin liner, distribute prepared batter into the cups and then bake for 18 minutes until the top has turned golden-brown and muffins pass the skewer test (if the skewer comes out clean from the center of muffins).

4. When done, let muffins cool in the tray for 10 minutes, then take them out and serve.

Nutrition Information Per Serving

Calories – 209

Fat – 13 g

Protein – 6 g

Carbohydrates – 15 g

Fiber – 2 g

Cholesterol – 31 ml

Net Carbs – 17 g

Sodium – 168 mg

Potassium – 197 mg

Phosphorus – 98 mg

Corn Bread Muffins

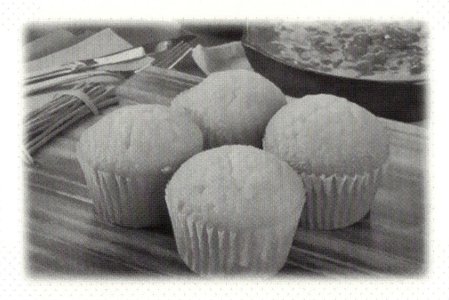

Preparation Time: 10 minutes/Cooking Time: 50 minutes/Servings – 12 muffins

Ingredients

- ❖ 1 cup yellow cornmeal
- ❖ 2 teaspoons baking powder
- ❖ 1 cup all-purpose white flour
- ❖ ¼ cup Splenda granulated sugar
- ❖ 2 tablespoons unsalted butter, melted
- ❖ ½ cup liquid egg substitute
- ❖ 1 cup of rice milk

Instructions

1. Switch on the oven, then set it to 400°F and let it preheat.

2. Meanwhile, take a large bowl, place cornmeal and flour in it, and stir in baking powder and sugar in it until mixed.

3. Take a separate bowl, add butter, pour in milk and egg substitute, whisk until blended and then stir in flour mixture until incorporated.

4. Take a twelve-cup muffin tray, line the cups with a muffin liner, distribute prepared batter into the cups and then bake for 20 minutes until the top has turned golden-brown and muffins passed the skewer test (if the skewer comes out clean from the center of muffins).

5. When done, let muffins cool in the tray for 5 minutes, then take them out and serve.

Nutrition Information Per Serving

Calories – 124

Fat – 3 g

Protein – 3 g

Carbohydrates – 23 g

Fiber – 1 g

Cholesterol – 5 ml

Net Carbs – 22 g

Sodium – 85 mg

Potassium – 40 mg

Phosphorus – 100 mg

Protein Booster Muffins with Blueberry

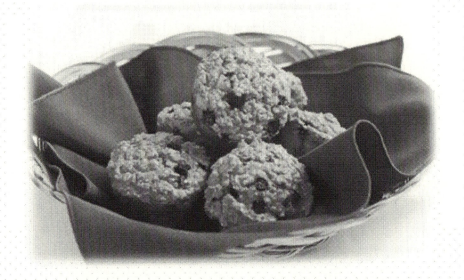

Preparation Time: 10 minutes/Cooking Time: 25 minutes/Servings – 12 muffins

Ingredients

- ❖ 1 cup rolled oats
- ❖ 1 cup blueberries, fresh
- ❖ 1 cup all-purpose white flour
- ❖ 1 1/3 cups whey protein powder
- ❖ ½ teaspoon salt
- ❖ 1 cup Greek yogurt, nonfat
- ❖ ¾ cup brown sugar
- ❖ ½ teaspoon baking soda

- ❖ ½ cup olive oil
- ❖ ¼ cup water
- ❖ 1 egg
- ❖ ½ teaspoon cream of tartar

Instructions

1. Switch on the oven, then set it to 350°F and let it preheat.

2. Meanwhile, take a large bowl, place oil in it, stir in yogurt, and then stir in sugar, oil, egg and water until combined.

3. Take a separate bowl, place flour in it, stir in remaining ingredients (except for berries), until mixed, then stir this mixture into the yogurt mixture until incorporated and fold in berries.

4. Take a twelve-cup muffin tray, line the cups with a muffin liner, distribute prepared batter into the cups and then bake for 25 minutes until the top has turned golden-brown and muffins passed the skewer test (if the skewer comes out clean from the center of muffins).

5. When done, let muffins cool in the tray for 5 minutes, then take them out and serve.

Nutrition Information Per Serving

Calories – 250

Fat – 10 g

Protein – 10 g

Carbohydrates – 30 g

Fiber – 1.3 g

Cholesterol – 31 ml

Net Carbs – 28.7 g

Sodium – 178 mg

Potassium – 136 mg

Phosphorus – 85 mg

Lunch

Baked Cauliflower and Broccoli Mac and Cheese

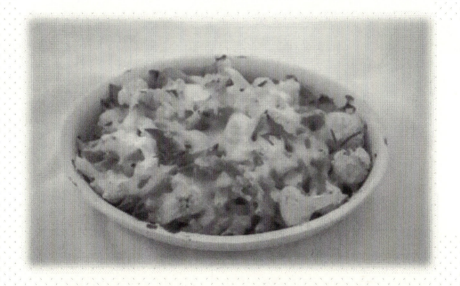

Preparation Time: 10 minutes/Cooking Time: 40 minutes/Servings – 8

Ingredients

- ❖ 12 ounces penne pasta, cooked
- ❖ 3 tablespoons all-purpose white flour
- ❖ 2 cups broccoli florets, steamed
- ❖ ½ cup white onion, chopped
- ❖ 2 cups cauliflower florets, steamed

- ❖ ¼ teaspoon minced garlic
- ❖ 2 tablespoons brown mustard
- ❖ 4 tablespoons unsalted butter
- ❖ ½ teaspoon ground black pepper
- ❖ ¼ teaspoon nutmeg
- ❖ 1 cup panko bread crumbs
- ❖ 1 cup Swiss cheese, shredded
- ❖ ½ cup parmesan cheese, shredded
- ❖ 1 cup white cheddar cheese, shredded
- ❖ 2 ½ cups rice drink

Instructions

1. Switch on the oven, then set it to 350°F and let it preheat.
2. Take a medium-sized pot, place it over medium heat, add 3 tablespoons butter and when it melts, add onion and garlic and cook for 4 minutes until tender.
3. Stir in flour, cook for 1 minute until thickened, and then stir in mustard.
4. Mix all the three cheeses, add 2/3 of the cheeses mixture, stir well until it has melted, remove the pot from heat, add pasta, broccoli and cauliflower florets and stir until well coated.
5. Take a 9-by-12 baking pan, grease it well, spoon in prepared pasta mixture, top with remaining cheese mixture, and then bake for 30 minutes.

6. Then melt the remaining butter, add bread crumbs, stir until mixed, cook for 2 minutes until golden, then top it over pasta mixture after 30 minutes and continue baking for 10 minutes until the top has turned brown.
7. Serve straight away.

Nutrition Information Per Serving

Calories – 442

Fat – 18 g

Protein – 18 g

Carbohydrates – 52 g

Fiber – 2.2 g

Cholesterol – 50 ml

Net Carbs – 49.8 g

Sodium – 308 mg

Potassium – 278 mg

Phosphorus – 315 mg

Caraway Cabbage and Rice

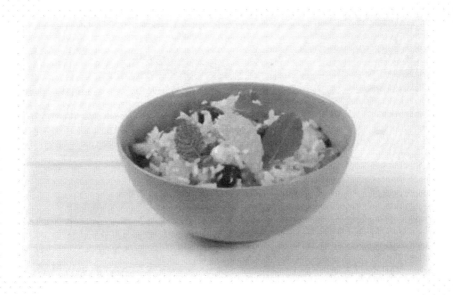

Preparation Time: 5 minutes/Cooking Time: 10 minutes/Servings – 2

Ingredients

- ❖ 1 cup of rice, cooked
- ❖ ¼ cup mandarin oranges
- ❖ 1 tablespoon white onion, chopped
- ❖ 1 cup cabbage, shredded
- ❖ ½ teaspoon caraway seed
- ❖ 1 tablespoon Worcestershire sauce
- ❖ ¼ cup water

Instructions

1. Take a frying pan, grease it with oil, place it over medium heat, add onion and cabbage and cook for 5 minutes until cabbage leaves wilted.

2. Stir in caraway seeds, Worcestershire sauce, and water, continue cooking for 3 minutes, add oranges and stir until rice until well combined.

3. Serve straight away.

Nutrition Information Per Serving

Calories – 142

Fat – 0 g

Protein – 3 g

Carbohydrates – 31 g

Fiber – 2.4 g

Cholesterol – 0 ml

Net Carbs – 28.6 g

Sodium – 101 mg

Potassium – 194 mg

Phosphorus – 51 mg

Gratin Pasta with Watercress and Chicken

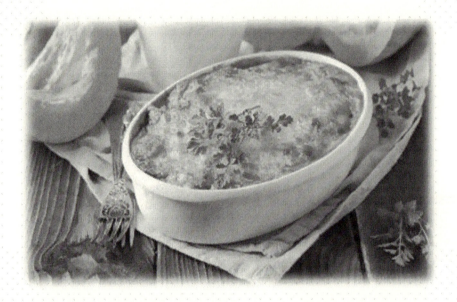

Preparation Time: 10 minutes/Cooking Time: 50 minutes/Servings – 4

Ingredients

- ❖ 2 cups pasta shells, cooked
- ❖ 1 cup chicken, shredded and cooked
- ❖ 1 small white onion, peeled and chopped
- ❖ 1 cup fresh watercress
- ❖ 1 teaspoon minced garlic
- ❖ ¼ teaspoon ground black pepper
- ❖ 1 tablespoon olive oil
- ❖ ½ cup Parmesan cheese, grated

❖ 1 2/3 cup béchamel sauce

Instructions

1. Take a medium-sized skillet pan, place it over medium heat, add oil and when hot, add onion and garlic, and cook for 4 minutes until sauted.

2. Then stir in chicken and watercress until mixed and continue cooking for 3 minutes until leaves of watercress have wilted.

3. Add pasta, pour in half of the béchamel sauce, mix until coated, and spoon the mixture into a greased baking dish.

4. Cover pasta with remaining béchamel sauce, sprinkle cheese on top and bake for 40 minutes until cheese has melts and pasta is bubbling.

5. Serve straight away.

Nutrition Information Per Serving

Calories – 345

Fat – 13 g

Protein – 19 g

Carbohydrates – 38 g

Fiber – 2.1 g

Cholesterol – 55 ml

Net Carbs – 35.9 g

Sodium – 437 mg

Potassium – 337 mg

Phosphorus – 248 mg

Orzo and Vegetables

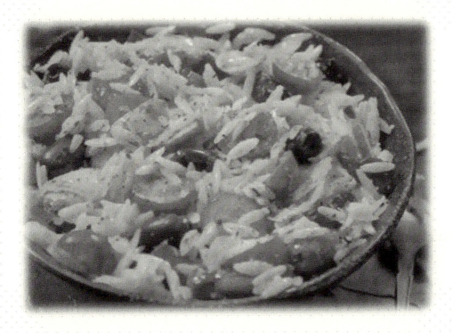

Preparation Time: 5 minutes/Cooking Time: 20 minutes/Servings – 6

Ingredients

- ❖ 1 medium carrot, peeled and shredded
- ❖ 1 small white onion, peeled and chopped
- ❖ 1 small zucchini, chopped
- ❖ ½ cup frozen green peas
- ❖ ½ teaspoon minced garlic
- ❖ ¼ teaspoon salt
- ❖ ¼ teaspoon ground black pepper
- ❖ 1 teaspoon curry powder
- ❖ 2 tablespoons olive oil

- ❖ ¼ cup Parmesan cheese, grated
- ❖ 3 cups chicken broth, low-sodium
- ❖ 2 tablespoons parsley, chopped
- ❖ 1 cup orzo pasta, uncooked

Instructions

1. Take a large skillet pan, place it over medium heat, add oil and when hot, add onion, garlic, carrot, and zucchini and cook for 5 minutes until sauted.
2. Stir in salt and curry powder, pour in the broth, stir until mixed and bring the mixture to a bowl.
3. Then stir in pasta, bring it to a boil, switch heat to medium-low level, and simmer for 10 minutes all the liquid has absorbed by the pasta.
4. Stir in remaining ingredients until mixed and cook for 3 minutes, or until hot.
5. Serve straight away.

Nutrition Information Per Serving

Calories – 176

Fat – 4 g

Protein – 10 g

Carbohydrates – 25 g

Fiber – 2.6 g

Cholesterol – 4 ml

Net Carbs – 22.4 g

Sodium – 193 mg

Potassium – 170 mg

Phosphorus – 68 mg

Lemon Rice with Vegetables

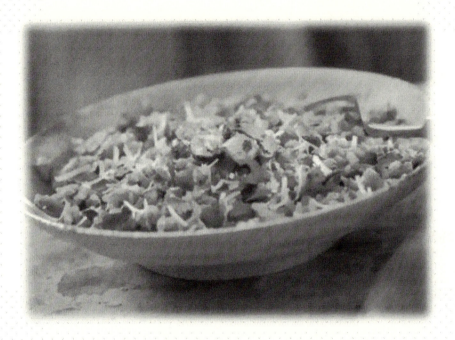

Preparation Time: 5 minutes/Cooking Time: 35

minutes/Servings – 5

Ingredients

- ❖ 10 tablespoons white rice, uncooked
- ❖ 1 ½ cups mushrooms, sliced
- ❖ ½ cup celery, sliced
- ❖ ¼ cup white onion, chopped
- ❖ 1/8 teaspoon ground black pepper
- ❖ 1/8 teaspoon dried thyme
- ❖ 1/8 teaspoon herb seasoning
- ❖ 1 teaspoon grated lemon zest

- ❖ 3 tablespoons unsalted margarine
- ❖ 2 tablespoons lemon juice
- ❖ 1 ¼ cups water

Instructions

1. Take a large skillet pan, place it over medium heat, add 1 ½ tablespoons margarine and when it melts, add onion and celery and cook for 5 minutes.
2. Season vegetables with lemon zest, black pepper, thyme, and herb seasoning, stir in water and lemon juice, bring to a boil, stir in rice, bring the mixture, then switch heat to medium-low level and simmer for 20 minutes until rice is tender.
3. Meanwhile, take a small-sized skillet pan, place it over medium heat, add remaining margarine and when it melts, add mushrooms and cook for 5 minutes until tender.
4. When the rice has cooked, stir cooked mushrooms in it and serve immediately.

Nutrition Information Per Serving

Calories – 183

Fat – 7 g

Protein – 3 g

Carbohydrates – 27 g

Fiber – 0.7 g

Cholesterol – 0 ml

Net Carbs – 26.3 g

Sodium – 13 mg

Potassium – 143 mg

Phosphorus – 37 mg

Chicken and Asparagus Pasta

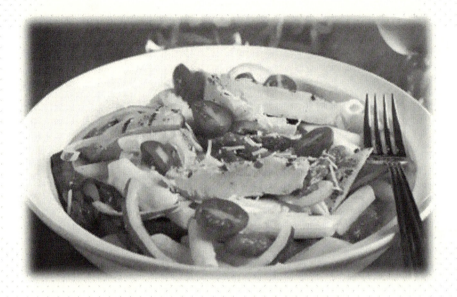

Preparation Time: 5 minutes/Cooking Time: 20 minutes/Servings – 8

Ingredients

❖ 8 ounces skinless chicken breasts, cubed

❖ 16 ounces penne pasta, cooked

❖ 1 pound asparagus spears, trimmed

❖ ½ teaspoon minced garlic

❖ ¼ teaspoon garlic powder

❖ ½ teaspoon ground black pepper

❖ 1 ½ teaspoons dried oregano

❖ 5 tablespoons olive oil

¼ cup feta cheese, crumbled
❖ ½ cup chicken broth, low-sodium

Instructions

1. Take a large skillet pan, place it over medium-high heat, add 3 tablespoons oil and when hot, add chicken cubes, stir in garlic powder and ¼ teaspoon black pepper and continue cooking for 5 minutes until cooked and browned.

2. When done, transfer chicken cubes to a plate lined with paper towels, then pour in chicken broth, add asparagus, season with oregano and remaining black pepper, and cook for 5 minutes until asparagus has steamed, covering the pan.

3. Then stir in chicken, cook for 3 minutes until warmed, stir in pasta, stir until mixed and cook for 5 minutes until hot, set aside until needed.

4. Drizzle with remaining oil, top with cheese, and serve.

Nutrition Information Per Serving

Calories – 376

Fat – 12 g

Protein – 18 g

Carbohydrates – 49 g

Fiber – 3 g

Cholesterol – 25 ml

Net Carbs – 46 g

Sodium – 110 mg

Potassium – 243 mg

Phosphorus – 193 mg

Hawaiian Rice

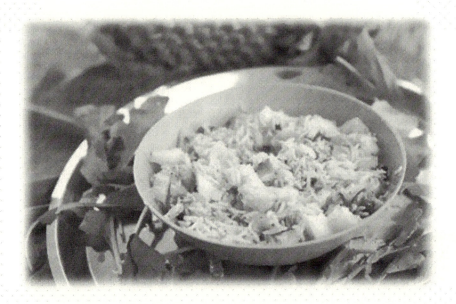

Preparation Time: 5 minutes/Cooking Time: 13 minutes/Servings – 6

Ingredients

- ❖ ½ cup pineapple tidbits, unsweetened
- ❖ ½ cup red bell pepper, chopped
- ❖ ½ cup mushrooms, chopped
- ❖ 1 teaspoon ginger root, minced
- ❖ ½ cup bean sprouts
- ❖ ½ tablespoon soy sauce, reduced-sodium
- ❖ ¼ teaspoon salt
- ❖ 2 cups brown rice, cooked

Instructions

1. Take a frying pan, spray it with oil, place it over medium heat and when hot, add all the vegetables and cook for 5 minutes until sauted.

2. Then stir in ginger and pineapple, drizzle with soy sauce, season with salt and cook for 3 minutes, or until hot.

3. Stir in rice until well mixed, cook for 3 minutes until hot, and then serve.

Nutrition Information Per Serving

Calories – 97

Fat – 1 g

Protein – 2 g

Carbohydrates – 20 g

Fiber – 1.8 g

Cholesterol – 0 ml

Net Carbs – 18.2 g

Sodium – 135 mg

Potassium – 181 mg

Phosphorus – 67 mg

Mexican Rice

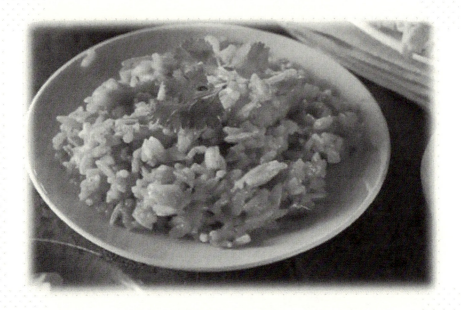

Preparation Time: 10 minutes/Cooking Time: 30 minutes/Servings – 6

Ingredients

- ❖ ¼ cup white onion, chopped
- ❖ ½ teaspoon minced garlic
- ❖ ¼ teaspoon salt
- ❖ ¼ cup canola oil
- ❖ ¼ cup tomato sauce, low-sodium
- ❖ 3 cups of water
- ❖ 1 cup white rice, uncooked

Instructions

1. Take a medium-sized skillet pan, place it over medium-high heat, add oil and when hot, add rice and cook for 5 minutes until browned.

2. Then add onion and garlic, stir until mixed, and cook for 3 minutes, or until tender.

3. Season with salt, pour in tomato sauce and water, stir until mixed, simmer for 20 minutes until rice has cooked, covering the pan.

4. Serve straight away.

Nutrition Information Per Serving

Calories – 194

Fat – 10 g

Protein – 2 g

Carbohydrates – 24 g

Fiber – 0.5 g

Cholesterol – 0 ml

Net Carbs – 23.5 g

Sodium – 94 mg

Potassium – 77 mg

Phosphorus – 41 mg

Shrimp Fried Rice

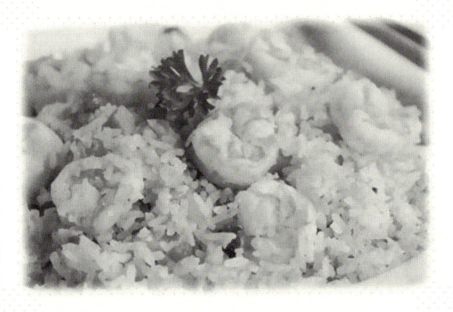

Preparation Time: 5 minutes/Cooking Time: 20 minutes/Servings – 4

Ingredients

- ❖ 4 cups white rice, cooked
- ❖ ½ cup small frozen shrimp, cooked
- ❖ ¾ cup white onion, chopped
- ❖ 1 cup frozen peas and carrots
- ❖ 3 tablespoons scallions, chopped
- ❖ ½ teaspoon minced garlic
- ❖ 1 tablespoon ginger root, grated
- ❖ ¼ teaspoon salt
- ❖ ¾ teaspoon ground black pepper

- ❖ 5 tablespoons peanut oil
- ❖ 4 eggs

Instructions

1. Take a large skillet pan, place it over medium-high heat, add 1 tablespoon peanut oil and when hot, add onion, season with ½ teaspoon black pepper, and cook for 2 minutes, or until onions are tender.

2. Stir in scallions, ginger, and garlic, cook for 1 minute, add shrimps, stir until mixed, cook for 2 minutes until hot, then stir in carrots and peas and cook for 2 minutes until hot.

3. When done, transfer shrimps and vegetable mixture to a bowl, cover with a lid and set aside until required.

4. Return the skillet pan over medium heat, add 2 tablespoons oil, beat the eggs, pour it into the pan, cook for 3 minutes until eggs are scrambled to desired level and then transfer eggs to the bowl containing shrimps and vegetables.

5. Add remaining 1 tablespoon oil and when hot, add rice, stir until well coated, and cook for 2 minutes until hot.

6. Then season rice with salt and remaining black pepper, cook for 2 minutes, don't stir, then add eggs, shrimps, and vegetables, stir until mixed and cook for 3 minutes until hot.

7. Serve straight away.

Nutrition Information Per Serving

Calories – 421

Fat – 16 g

Protein – 16 g

Carbohydrates – 53 g

Fiber – 2.5 g

Cholesterol – 244 ml

Net Carbs – 50.5 g

Sodium – 271 mg

Potassium – 285 mg

Phosphorus – 218 mg

Vegetarian Egg Fried Rice

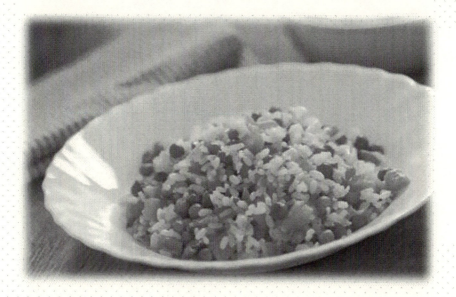

Preparation Time: 5 minutes/Cooking Time: 18

minutes/Servings – 6

Ingredients

- ❖ 4 cups white rice, cooked
- ❖ 1 cup diced tofu, extra-firm, drained
- ❖ ½ cup green onion, chopped
- ❖ 1 cup white onion, diced
- ❖ 1 cup fresh carrots, sliced
- ❖ ½ cup green peas
- ❖ 1 tablespoon ginger root, grated
- ❖ 1 teaspoon minced garlic
- ❖ ¼ teaspoon mustard powder
- ❖ ½ cup cilantro, chopped

- ❖ 3 tablespoons canola oil
- ❖ 1 tablespoon soy sauce, reduced-sodium
- ❖ 6 eggs, beaten

Instructions

1. Take a large skillet pan, place it over medium heat, add oil and when hot, add beaten eggs and cook the omelet for 3 minutes until eggs are cooked to the desired level.

2. Transfer omelet to a cutting board, let it cool for 5 minutes, and chop it, set aside until needed.

3. Add oil in the pan and when hot, add all the vegetables, stir in tofu, garlic, and ginger, season with mustard, cook for 5 minutes until carrots have softened.

4. Stir in rice and chopped eggs, drizzle with soy sauce, stir until well mixed and remove the pan from heat.

5. Garnish rice with green onion and cilantro and then serve.

Nutrition Information Per Serving

Calories – 343

Fat – 15 g

Protein – 15 g

Carbohydrates – 37 g

Fiber – 3.2 g

Cholesterol – 212 ml

Net Carbs – 33.8 g

Sodium – 238 mg

Potassium – 350 mg

Phosphorus – 230 mg

Autumn Orzo Salad

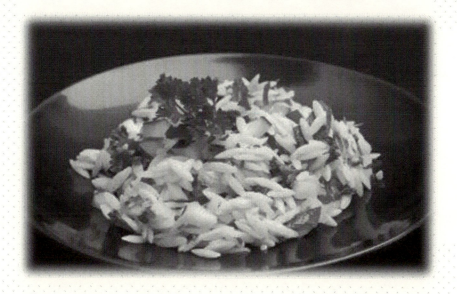

Preparation Time: 35 minutes/Cooking Time: 0 minutes/Servings – 4

Ingredients

- ❖ 1 medium apple, cored and diced
- ❖ ¾ cups orzo, cooked
- ❖ ¼ teaspoon ground black pepper
- ❖ 1 tablespoon fresh basil, chopped
- ❖ 2 tablespoons lemon juice
- ❖ 2 tablespoons olive oil
- ❖ 2 tablespoons almonds, sliced and blanched

Instructions

1. Take a medium-sized bowl, add all the ingredients in it (except for almonds), and stir until incorporated.

2. Take a baking dish, place prepared mixture in it, and place in the refrigerator for 30 minutes until chilled.

3. When ready to eat, garnish with almonds and serve.

Nutrition Information Per Serving

Calories – 227

Fat – 9 g

Protein – 5 g

Carbohydrates – 29 g

Fiber – 2.5 g

Cholesterol – 0 ml

Net Carbs – 26.5 g

Sodium – 2 mg

Potassium – 126 mg

Phosphorus – 62 mg

Blackened Shrimp and Pineapple Salad

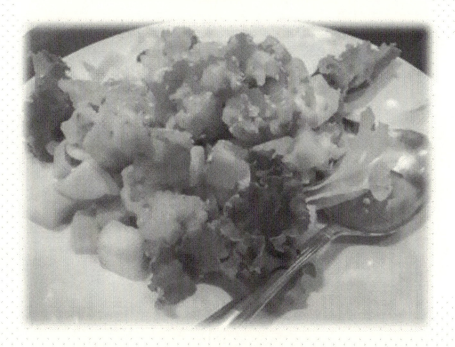

Preparation Time: 10 minutes/Cooking Time: 8 minutes/Servings – 2

Ingredients

- ❖ 2 cups romaine lettuce, diced
- ❖ ½ of medium red bell pepper, sliced
- ❖ 1 ½ cups pineapple chunks
- ❖ ¼ cup corn kernels
- ❖ 14 large shrimp, peeled and deveined
- ❖ 1 tablespoon blackening seasoning, low-sodium
- ❖ ¼ teaspoon ground black pepper

- ❖ 1 tablespoon unsalted butter
- ❖ 1 tablespoon rice vinegar, unseasoned
- ❖ 1 tablespoon olive oil

Instructions

1. Prepare the shrimps by sprinkling them with blackening seasoning.

2. Take a skillet pan, place it over medium-high heat, add butter and when it melts, add prepared shrimps and cook for 3 minutes per side, or until curled.

3. Transfer shrimps to a plate lined with paper towels and set aside until cooled.

4. Prepare the salad by placing all the vegetables in a large salad bowl, add corn and pineapple, season with black pepper, drizzle with vinegar and oil and toss until well mixed.

5. Top the salad with the shrimps and serve.

Nutrition Information Per Serving

Calories – 260

Fat – 14 g

Protein – 13 g

Carbohydrates – 20 g

Fiber – 4.5 g

Cholesterol – 90 ml

Net Carbs – 15.5 g

Sodium – 340 mg

Potassium – 468 mg

Phosphorus – 150 mg

Green Pepper Slaw

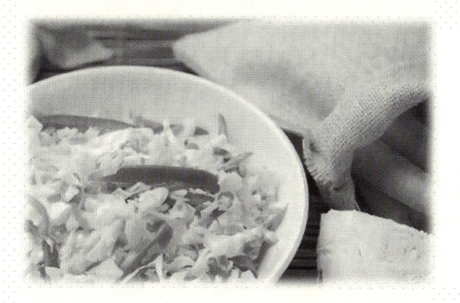

Preparation Time: 5 minutes/Cooking Time: 0 minutes

Servings – 12/

Ingredients

- ❖ 2 medium carrots, peeled and chopped
- ❖ 1 small head of cabbage, chopped
- ❖ 1 medium green bell pepper, cored and chopped
- ❖ 2 teaspoons celery seed
- ❖ ½ cup Splenda granulated sugar
- ❖ ½ cup apple cider vinegar
- ❖ ½ cup water

Instructions

1. Take a salad bowl, place carrot, cabbage, and bell pepper in it and mix well until combined.

2. Whisk together celery seeds, sugar, vinegar, and water until blended, drizzle it over the salad and toss until mixed.

3. Serve straight away.

Nutrition Information Per Serving

Calories – 76

Fat – 0 g

Protein – 1 g

Carbohydrates – 18 g

Fiber – 1 g

Cholesterol – 0 ml

Net Carbs – 17 g

Sodium – 9 mg

Potassium – 108 mg

Phosphorus – 13 mg

Italian Chicken Salad

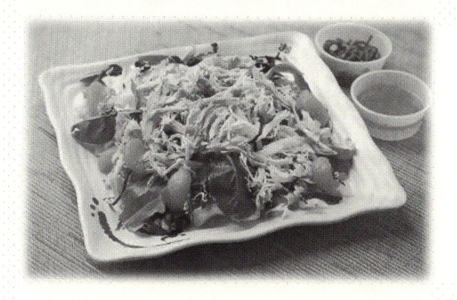

Preparation Time: 1 hour and 10 minutes/Cooking Time:
0 minutes/Servings – 4

Ingredients

- ❖ 4 chicken breasts, cooked, ½-inch cubed
- ❖ 2 cups grilled summer squash, sliced
- ❖ ¼ cup sweet onion, chopped
- ❖ 1 medium orange bell pepper, cored and chopped
- ❖ 2 cups baby arugula
- ❖ 6 sprigs of parsley, leaves chopped
- ❖ 1/8 teaspoon cayenne pepper
- ❖ ¼ cup lemon juice
- ❖ ½ cup mayonnaise

Instructions

1. Prepare the dressing by placing mayonnaise in a bowl, add parsley, season with cayenne pepper, drizzle with lemon juice, and whisk until combined.

2. Place chicken cubes in a salad bowl, add remaining ingredients, except for arugula, stir until mixed, then drizzle with prepared dressing and toss until well coated.

3. Place the salad bowl in the refrigerator and chill for 1 hour and then serve the salad with arugula.

Nutrition Information Per Serving

Calories – 421

Fat – 29 g

Protein – 30 g

Carbohydrates – 10 g

Fiber – 2.2 g

Cholesterol – 80 ml

Net Carbs – 7.8 g

Sodium – 256 mg

Potassium – 670 mg

Phosphorus – 270 mg

Cranberries and Couscous Salad

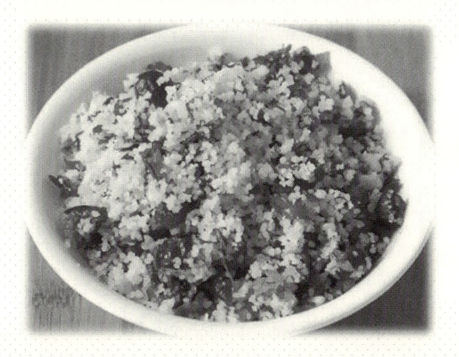

Preparation Time: 10 minutes/Cooking Time: 0 minutes/Servings – 10

Ingredients

- ❖ 1 cup dried cranberries, sweetened
- ❖ ½ cup green onion, chopped
- ❖ 1 ½ cups couscous, cooked
- ❖ ½ cup celery, chopped
- ❖ ½ cup cucumber, chopped
- ❖ 2 teaspoons lemon zest

- ❖ ½ teaspoon ground cumin
- ❖ 1 tablespoon parsley, chopped
- ❖ ¼ teaspoon ground cayenne pepper
- ❖ ¼ cup lemon juice
- ❖ 1 tablespoon olive oil

Instructions

1. Take a large bowl, add couscous in it, drizzle with lemon juice, season with all the spices, and stir until combined.
2. Add remaining ingredients, stir until mixed, and then serve.

Nutrition Information Per Serving

Calories – 158

Fat – 2 g

Protein – 4 g

Carbohydrates – 31 g

Fiber – 2.5 g

Cholesterol – 0 ml

Net Carbs – 28.5 g

Sodium – 11 mg

Potassium – 103 mg

Phosphorus – 55 mg

Tuna Salad

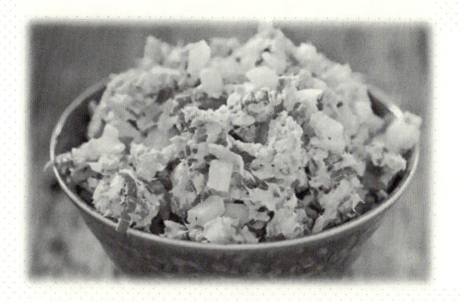

Preparation Time: 10 minutes/Cooking Time: 0 minutes/Servings – 4

Ingredients

- ❖ ½ of large apple, cored and chopped
- ❖ 15 ounces tuna, packed in water, unsalted
- ❖ ½ of small white onion, peeled and chopped
- ❖ 1 celery stalk, chopped
- ❖ 1/8 teaspoon salt
- ❖ 1/8 teaspoon ground black pepper
- ❖ 3 tablespoons mayonnaise
- ❖ Lettuce for serving

Instructions

1. Prepare the salad by taking a bowl, place tuna in it, add remaining ingredients in it (except for lettuce), and stir until mixed.

2. Place the salad on the lettuce and serve.

Nutrition Information Per Serving

Calories – 202

Fat – 9 g

Protein – 27 g

Carbohydrates – 3 g

Fiber – 0.8 g

Cholesterol – 36 ml

Net Carbs – 2.2 g

Sodium – 188 mg

Potassium – 318 mg

Phosphorus – 183 mg

Mixed Berry and Fruit Salad

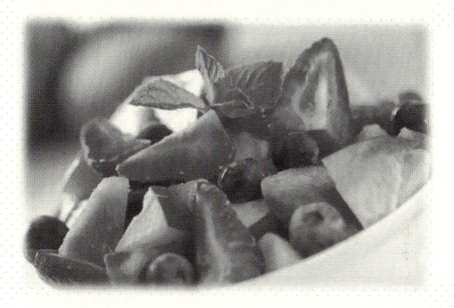

Preparation Time: 1 hour and 5 minutes/Cooking Time: 0 minutes/Servings – 4

Ingredients

- ❖ 2 cups fresh strawberries, quartered
- ❖ 10 leaves of fresh basil
- ❖ 1 cup fresh blueberries
- ❖ 1 tablespoon Splenda granulated sugar
- ❖ 2 tablespoons white balsamic vinegar
- ❖ ¼ cup almond and coconut milk blend

Instructions

1. Take a large bowl, pour in the milk, and stir in sugar and vinegar until combined.

2. Add all the berries, toss well until combined, cover the bowl and place it into the refrigerator for 1 hour until chilled.

3. When ready to eat, stir basil into the salad and serve.

Nutrition Information Per Serving

Calories – 65

Fat – 1 g

Protein – 1 g

Carbohydrates – 13 g

Fiber – 2.4 g

Cholesterol – 0 ml

Net Carbs – 10.6 g

Sodium – 10 mg

Potassium – 160 mg

Phosphorus – 25 mg

Roasted Vegetable Salad

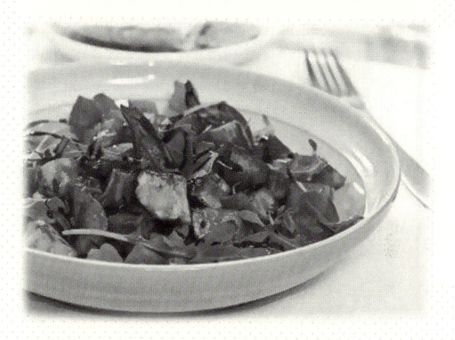

Preparation Time: 10 minutes/Cooking Time: 35 minutes/Servings – 8

Ingredients

- ❖ 6 cups baby leaf lettuce, chopped
- ❖ 1 small head cauliflower, cut into florets
- ❖ 5 medium carrots, peeled, 2-inch diced
- ❖ ½ cup pomegranate seeds
- ❖ 1 large turnip, peeled and diced
- ❖ 1 medium white onion, peeled and diced
- ❖ ¼ teaspoon ground black pepper
- ❖ 1 tablespoon Italian seasoning blend

- ❖ ¼ teaspoon yellow mustard
- ❖ ¼ teaspoon salt
- ❖ 1 ½ tablespoons maple syrup
- ❖ 3 tablespoons rice vinegar, unseasoned
- ❖ 6 tablespoons olive oil

Instructions

1. Switch on the oven, then set it to 425°F and let it preheat.

2. Meanwhile, take a large bowl, place all the vegetables in it, except for lettuce, season with Italian seasoning, drizzle with 3 tablespoons oil and toss until coated.

3. Take a baking sheet, place all the vegetables in it, and bake for 35 minutes until tender, turning halfway.

4. While vegetables are baking, prepare the dressing by placing remaining oil in a small bowl and whisk in salt, black pepper, mustard, vinegar, and maple syrup until combined.

5. When vegetables have roasted, transfer them to a salad bowl, add lettuce, drizzle with prepared dressing and toss until well coated.

6. Top the salad with pomegranate seeds and then serve.

Nutrition Information Per Serving

Calories – 160

Fat – 11 g

Protein – 2 g

Carbohydrates – 13 g

Fiber – 3.1 g

Cholesterol – 0 ml

Net Carbs – 9.9 g

Sodium – 134 mg

Potassium – 378 mg

Phosphorus – 53 mg

Chicken Pita Pizza

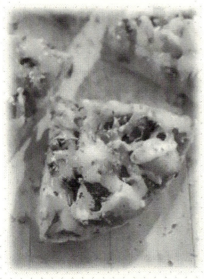

Preparation Time: 5 minutes

Cooking Time: 12 minutes

Servings – 2

Ingredients

- ❖ 4 ounces chicken, cooked and cubed
- ❖ 1/8 teaspoon garlic powder
- ❖ ¼ cup purple onion, chopped
- ❖ 3 tablespoons barbecue sauce, low-sodium
- ❖ 2 tablespoons feta cheese, crumbled
- ❖ 2 pita breads, about 6 ½ inches

Instructions

1. Switch on the oven, then set it to 350°F and let it preheat.
2. Take a baking sheet, spray it with oil, place pitas on it, spread 1 ½ tablespoon of sauce on each pita, then scatter with onions and chicken.
3. Sprinkle cheese and garlic powder on top of pitas and bake for 12 minutes until cooked.
4. Serve straight away.

Nutrition Information Per Serving

Calories – 320

Fat – 9 g

Protein – 23 g

Carbohydrates – 37 g

Fiber – 2.4 g

Cholesterol – 55 ml

Net Carbs – 34.6 g

Sodium – 523 mg

Potassium – 255 mg

Phosphorus – 221 mg

Cauliflower Steak Sandwiches

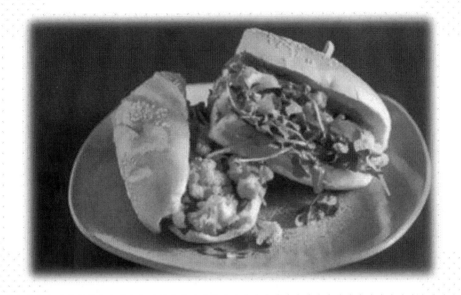

Preparation Time: 15 minutes/Cooking Time: 40 minutes/Servings – 4

Ingredients

- ❖ 1 medium head cauliflower
- ❖ ¼ cup chopped red onion
- ❖ ¼ teaspoon garlic powder
- ❖ ¼ teaspoon ground black pepper
- ❖ ¼ teaspoon onion powder
- ❖ 1/8 teaspoon salt
- ❖ 4 teaspoons mustard
- ❖ 3 tablespoons olive oil
- ❖ 4 lettuce leaves

- ❖ 2 tablespoons and 2 teaspoons mayonnaise
- ❖ 4 hamburger buns

Instructions

1. Switch on the oven, then set it to 400°F and then let it preheat.
2. Prepare the cauliflower steaks by cutting four 1-inch thick slices and reserve the rest of cauliflower for later use.
3. Place oil in a small bowl, stir in salt, black pepper, onion powder, and garlic powder until mixed, and brush half of this mixture on both sides of cauliflower steaks.
4. Place the seasoned cauliflower steak on a baking sheet lined with parchment paper and bake for 40 minutes until cooked, flipping, and turning cauliflower halfway.
5. When done, sandwich a cauliflower steak into each bun, spread 2 teaspoon mayonnaise on each steak, sprinkle with 1 teaspoon mustard, top with some slices of onion and lettuce and then serve.

Nutrition Information Per Serving

Calories – 305	Cholesterol – 4 ml
Fat – 19 g	Net Carbs – 24.4 g
Protein – 7 g	Sodium – 430 mg
Carbohydrates – 28 g	Potassium – 427 mg
Fiber – 3.6 g	Phosphorus – 107 mg

Chicken Wraps

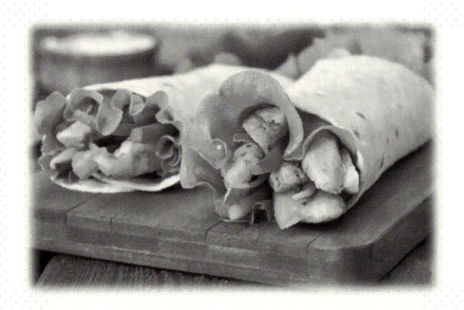

Preparation Time: 10 minutes/Cooking Time: 0 minutes/Servings – 4

Ingredients

- ❖ 8 ounces cooked chicken, low-sodium
- ❖ 1 stalk celery, diced
- ❖ ½ of medium red bell pepper, cored and diced
- ❖ ½ teaspoon onion powder
- ❖ 1 medium carrot, peeled and diced
- ❖ ¼ cup mayonnaise, low-fat
- ❖ 2 lavash, whole-wheat tortillas

Instructions

1. Place mayonnaise in a bowl, stir in onion powder until mixed and then spread 2 tablespoons of this mixture onto each bread.

2. Take a medium bowl, place all the vegetables in it, toss until mixed and distribute vegetables evenly on one side of each tortilla.

3. Roll the tortillas, then cut in half, secure with a toothpick and serve.

Nutrition Information Per Serving

Calories – 260

Fat – 9 g

Protein – 17 g

Carbohydrates – 27 g

Fiber – 3 g

Cholesterol – 42 ml

Net Carbs – 24 g

Sodium – 462 mg

Potassium – 215 mg

Phosphorus – 103 mg

Salmon Sandwiches

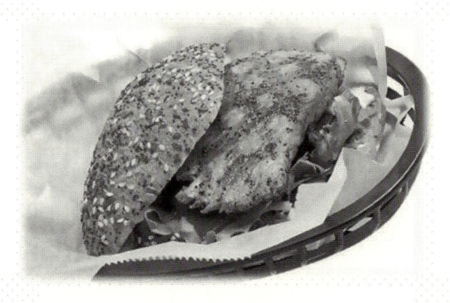

Preparation Time: 10 minutes/Cooking Time: 15 minutes/Servings – 4

Ingredients

- ❖ 4 salmon fillets, each about 4 ounces
- ❖ ½ cup roasted red peppers, diced
- ❖ 1 cup arugula
- ❖ ½ teaspoon lemon-and-pepper seasoning, salt-free
- ❖ 1 tablespoon lime juice¼ cup chipotle mayonnaise
- ❖ 2 tablespoons olive oil
- ❖ 4 slices of sourdough bread

Instructions

1. Prepare the grill: set the grill, brush its grilling rack with oil, and let it preheat over medium-high heat.

2. Brush salmon fillets with 1 tablespoon oil, place them on the grill, and cook for 15 minutes, or until fork tender.

3. When salmon has grilled, transfer it to a plate, cover the plate with foil, let it rest for 5 minutes, and then remove the skin.

4. Meanwhile, place remaining oil in a small bowl, whisk in lemon-and-pepper seasoning, and lemon juice until mixed, then brush this mixture on both sides of bread slices and grill them for 2 minutes per side until toasted, set aside until required.

5. Assemble sandwiches: spread chipotle mayonnaise on one side of the toasted slice, top with grilled salmon, arugula and red pepper and then serve.

Nutrition Information Per Serving

Calories – 382   Cholesterol – 68 ml

Fat – 22 g   Net Carbs – 19 g

Protein – 26 g   Sodium – 384 mg

Carbohydrates – 20 g   Potassium – 640 mg

Fiber – 1 g   Phosphorus – 268 mg

Mexican Chicken Pizza

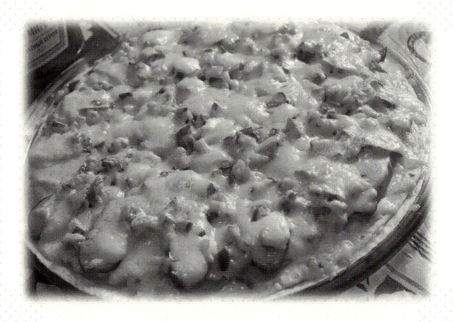

Preparation Time: 10 minutes/Cooking Time: 12 minutes/Servings – 4

Ingredients

- ❖ 2 cups roasted chicken breast, diced
- ❖ ½ cup red bell peppers, diced
- ❖ 1 cup kernel corn, salt-free
- ❖ ¼ cup onion, diced
- ❖ 2 tablespoons lime juice
- ❖ 4 teaspoons chopped cilantro
- ❖ ½ teaspoon minced garlic
- ❖ ½ cup shredded Monterey Jack cheese
- ❖ 4 flour tortillas, each about 6 inches

Instructions

1. Switch on the oven, then set it to 350°F and let it preheat.

2. Then place tortillas onto a greased baking sheet and bake for 10 minutes until its edges are light brown.

3. Meanwhile, take a large skillet pan, place it over medium-high heat, grease it with oil and when hot, add corn and cook for 1 minute until corn is lightly charred.

4. Add chicken, onion, red peppers and garlic, cook for 2 minutes until hot, remove the pan from heat and then stir in lime juice until mixed.

5. When tortillas have baked, place ¾ cup of the chicken mixture on top of each tortilla, then top with 2 tablespoons of cheese and continue baking for 2 minutes, or until cheese has melted.

6. When done, sprinkle cilantro over pizza and serve.

Nutrition Information Per Serving

Calories – 309

Fat – 9 g

Protein – 26 g

Carbohydrates – 31 g

Fiber – 2.1 g

Cholesterol – 59 ml

Net Carbs – 28.9 g

Sodium – 253 mg

Potassium – 329 mg

Phosphorus – 250 mg

Shrimp Po Boy Sandwiches

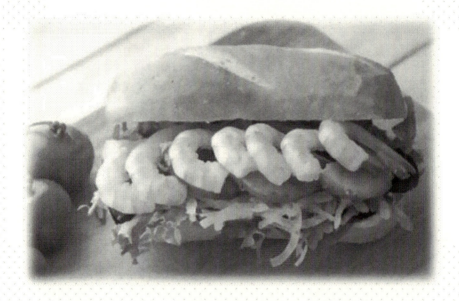

Preparation Time: 10 minutes/Cooking Time: 10 minutes/Servings – 2

Ingredients

- ❖ 1 cup iceberg lettuce, shredded
- ❖ 1 small Roma tomato, sliced
- ❖ 4 ounces of frozen cooked shrimp, thawed
- ❖ 3 tablespoons all-purpose white flour
- ❖ ¼ teaspoon baking powder
- ❖ 1 teaspoon Cajun seasoning, salt-free
- ❖ ¼ teaspoon ground black pepper
- ❖ ½ teaspoon Tabasco sauce
- ❖ ½ of egg

- ❖ 4 teaspoons mayonnaise
- ❖ ¼ cup beer
- ❖ 4 cups olive oil
- ❖ 1 French baguette, about 12 inches long
- ❖ 1 ounce low-sodium sweet pickles, chopped

Instructions

1. Pat dry shrimps, place them in a bowl, sprinkle with Cajun seasoning, and toss until coated.

2. Place half egg in a large bowl, add flour, black pepper, and baking powder in it, pour in beet and whisk until smooth batter comes together.

3. Add shrimps into the batter and toss until well coated.

4. Take a skillet pan, place it over medium-high heat, pour in oil, then bring it to 375°F, add shrimps in it in a single layer and cook for 5 minutes, or until golden-brown.

5. When done, transfer shrimps to a plate lined with paper towels and fry the remaining shrimps in the same manner.

6. Prepare the sandwich: cut the bread in half, each piece about 6 inches long, then slice it open, spread mayonnaise in the inner side, and then fill with tomato, lettuce, and pickles.

7. Distribute fried shrimps in the sandwich evenly, sprinkle with Tabasco sauce, close the sandwich, and serve.

Nutrition Information Per Serving

Calories – 504

Fat – 24 g

Protein – 24 g

Carbohydrates – 48 g

Fiber – 2.8 g

Cholesterol – 157 ml

Net Carbs – 45.2 g

Sodium – 529 mg

Potassium – 422 mg

Phosphorus – 270 mg

Tuna Salad Bagel

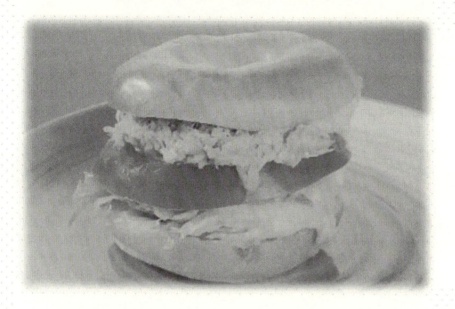

Preparation Time: 5 minutes/Cooking Time: 0
minutes/Servings – 1

Ingredients

- ❖ 1 medium bagel, about 2 ounces
- ❖ 1 leaf of lettuce
- ❖ 1 tablespoon onion, chopped
- ❖ ½ cup tuna,water-packed, low-sodium
- ❖ 1 tablespoon celery, chopped
- ❖ 1 tablespoon mayonnaise, reduced-calorie

Instructions

1. Drain the tuna, break it into pieces, then place it in a bowl, add onion, celery, and mayonnaise and stir until mixed.

2. Take a bagel, line it with a lettuce leaf, spread tuna mixture on it, and serve.

Nutrition Information Per Serving

Calories – 290

Fat – 7 g

Protein – 25 g

Carbohydrates – 32 g

Fiber – 2.5 g

Cholesterol – 22 ml

Net Carbs – 29.5 g

Sodium – 475 mg

Potassium – 320 mg

Phosphorus – 175 mg

Turkey Meatball Gyros

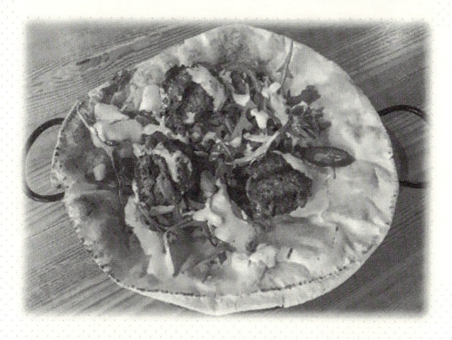

Preparation Time: 10 minutes/Cooking Time: 15 minutes/Servings – 8

Ingredients

- ❖ 4 pita breads, whole-wheat, each about the 6 ½ inches in diameter
- ❖ 1 pound ground turkey
- ❖ 1 cup baby lettuce mix, chopped
- ❖ 1 teaspoon minced garlic
- ❖ ½ teaspoon ground cumin
- ❖ 1/3 cup panko breadcrumbs
- ❖ 1 egg

- ❖ 4 tablespoons feta cheese, crumbled

Tzatziki Sauce
- ❖ ½ cup diced cucumber
- ❖ 1 cup Greek yogurt, nonfat
- ❖ ½ teaspoon garlic powder
- ❖ ¼ teaspoon ground black pepper
- ❖ ½ teaspoon dried dill
- ❖ 1 tablespoon lemon juice

Instructions

1. Switch on the oven, then set it to 425°F and let it preheat.

2. Meanwhile, prepare the tzatziki sauce by placing cucumber in a bowl, add remaining ingredients for the sauce, stir until combined, cover the bowl and refrigerate until required.

3. Take a large bowl, place ground meat in it, season with garlic powder, black pepper, and cumin, add breadcrumbs and egg, stir until well-combined and then shape the mixture into 32 balls.

4. Take a cookie sheet, grease it with oil, place meatballs on it and bake for 15 minutes, or until meatballs are golden-brown, and their internal temperature reaches 165°F, turning meatballs halfway.

5. When done, remove the cookie sheet from the oven and let meatballs rest for 10 minutes.

6. Then cut each pita bread in half, spread 2 ½ tablespoons of prepared tzatziki sauce onto one side of each pita half, top with four baked meatballs, then top with 2 tablespoons lettuce and ½ tablespoon feta cheese and serve.

Nutrition Information Per Serving

Calories – 229

Fat – 7 g

Protein – 20 g

Carbohydrates – 23 g

Fiber – 2.2 g

Cholesterol – 68 ml

Net Carbs – 20.8 g

Sodium – 274 mg

Potassium – 286 mg

Phosphorus – 246 mg

Dinner

Meatloaf

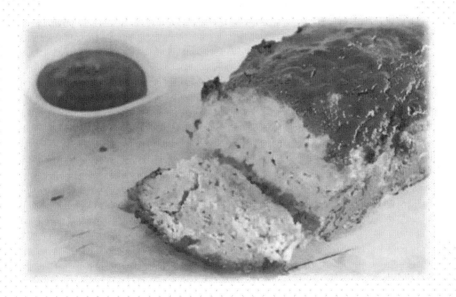

Preparation Time: 10 minutes/Cooking Time: 50 minutes/Servings – 6

Ingredients

- ❖ 1 pound lean ground beef
- ❖ 2 tablespoons white onion, chopped
- ❖ ¼ teaspoon ground black pepper
- ❖ 1 tablespoon brown sugar
- ❖ 1 egg
- ❖ 1/3 cup catsup

- ❖ ½ teaspoon apple cider vinegar
- ❖ 2 tablespoons milk, low-fat
- ❖ 1 teaspoon water
- ❖ 20 squares saltine-type crackers, unsalted tops, crushed

Instructions

1. Switch on the oven, then set it to 350°F and let it preheat.
2. Take a large bowl, place beef, onion, and crackers in it, sprinkle with black pepper, pour in egg and milk, and stir until well combined.
3. Take a loaf pan, place beef mixture in it and bake for 40 minutes until cooked.
4. Meanwhile, prepare the sauce by placing catsup in a small bowl and whisk in vinegar, sugar and water until combined.
5. When meatloaf has baked, cover its top with the prepared sauce and bake for 10 minutes until the top is glazed, and the internal temperature of meatloaf reaches 160°F.
6. When done, let meatloaf cool for 5 minutes, then take it out, slice it into six pieces, and serve.

Nutrition Information Per Serving

Calories – 205

Fat – 9 g

Protein – 17 g

Carbohydrates – 14 g

Fiber – 0.5 g

Cholesterol – 84 ml

Net Carbs – 13.5 g

Sodium – 299 mg

Potassium – 255 mg

Phosphorus – 147 mg

Apple Spice Pork Chops

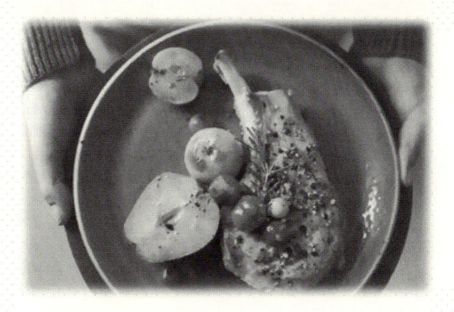

Preparation Time: 10 minutes/Cooking Time: 10 minutes/Servings – 4

Ingredients

- ❖ 2 medium apples: peeled, cored, sliced
- ❖ 1 pound pork chops
- ❖ ¼ teaspoon salt
- ❖ ¼ cup brown sugar
- ❖ ¼ teaspoon ground nutmeg
- ❖ ¼ teaspoon ground black pepper
- ❖ ¼ teaspoon cinnamon
- ❖ 2 tablespoons unsalted butter

Instructions

1. Switch on the broiler, let it preheat, then place pork chops in it and cook for 5 minutes per side until done.

2. Meanwhile, take a medium-sized skillet pan, place it over medium heat, add butter and when it melts, add apples, sprinkle with black pepper, salt, sugar, cinnamon, and nutmeg, stir well and cook for 8 minutes, or until apples are tender and the sauce has thickened to the desired level.

3. When done, spoon the applesauce over pork chops and serve.

Nutrition Information Per Serving

Calories – 306

Fat – 16 g

Protein – 22 g

Carbohydrates – 21 g

Fiber – 1.2 g

Cholesterol – 88 ml

Net Carbs – 19.8 g

Sodium – 192 mg

Potassium – 473 mg

Phosphorus – 194 mg

Beef Burritos

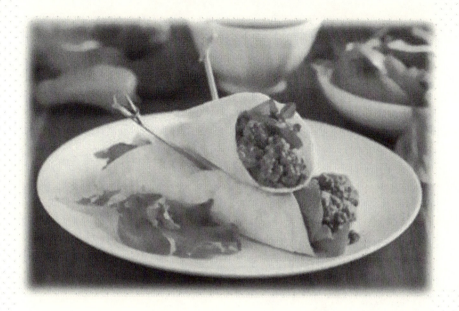

Preparation Time: 10 minutes/Cooking Time: 20 minutes/Servings – 6

Ingredients

- ❖ ¼ cup white onion, chopped
- ❖ ¼ cup green bell pepper, chopped
- ❖ 1 pound ground beef
- ❖ ¼ cup tomato puree, low-sodium
- ❖ ¼ teaspoon ground black pepper
- ❖ ¼ teaspoon ground cumin
- ❖ 6 flour tortillas, burrito size

Instructions

1. Take a skillet pan, place it over medium heat and when hot, add beef and cook for 5 to 8 minutes until browned.

2. Drain the excess fat, then transfer beef to a plate lined with paper towels and serve.

3. Return pan over medium heat, grease it with oil and when hot, add pepper and onion and cook for 5 minutes, or until softened.

4. Switch to low heat, return beef to the pan, season with black pepper and cumin, pour in tomato puree, stir until mixed and cook for 5 minutes until done.

5. Distribute beef mixture evenly on top of the tortilla, roll them in burrito style by folding both ends and then serve.

Nutrition Information Per Serving

Calories – 265

Fat – 9 g

Protein – 15 g

Carbohydrates – 31 g

Fiber – 1.6 g

Cholesterol – 37 ml

Net Carbs – 29.4 g

Sodium – 341 mg

Potassium – 302 mg

Phosphorus – 171 mg

Broccoli and Beef Stir-Fry

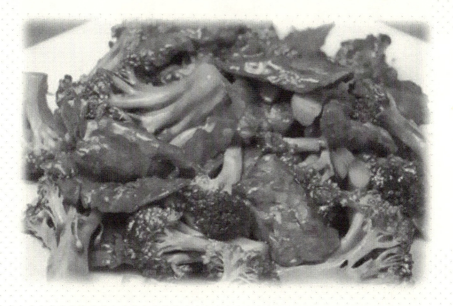

Preparation Time: 5 minutes/Cooking Time: 18 minutes/Servings – 4

Ingredients

- ❖ 12 ounces frozen broccoli, thawed
- ❖ 8 ounces sirloin beef, cut into thin strips
- ❖ 1 medium Roma tomato, chopped
- ❖ 1 teaspoon minced garlic
- ❖ 1 tablespoon cornstarch
- ❖ 2 tablespoons soy sauce, reduced-sodium
- ❖ ¼ cup chicken broth, low-sodium
- ❖ 2 tablespoons peanut oil
- ❖ 2 cups cooked brown rice

Instructions

1. Take a frying pan, place it over medium heat, add oil and when hot, add garlic and cook for 1 minute until fragrant.

2. Add vegetable blend, cook for 5 minutes, then transfer vegetable blend to a plate and set aside until needed.

3. Add beef strips into the pan, and then cook for 7 minutes until cooked to the desired level.

4. Prepare the sauce by putting cornstarch in a bowl, and then whisking in soy sauce and broth until well combined.

5. Returned vegetables to the pan, add tomatoes, drizzle with sauce, stir well until coated, and cook for 2 minutes until the sauce has thickened.

6. Serve with brown rice.

Nutrition Information Per Serving

Calories – 373

Fat – 17 g

Protein – 18 g

Carbohydrates – 37 g

Fiber – 5.1 g

Cholesterol – 42 ml

Net Carbs – 31.9 g

Sodium – 351 mg

Potassium – 555 mg

Phosphorus – 255 mg

Meatballs with Eggplant

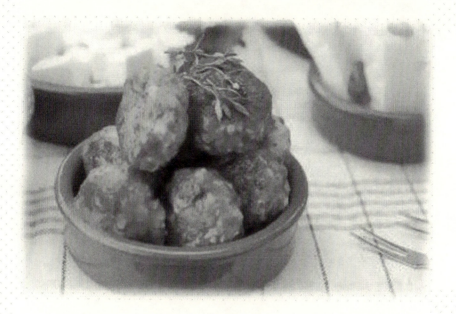

Preparation Time: 15 minutes/Cooking Time: 60 minutes/Servings – 6

Ingredients

- ❖ 1 pound ground beef
- ❖ ½ cup green bell pepper, chopped
- ❖ 2 medium eggplants, peeled and diced
- ❖ ½ teaspoon minced garlic
- ❖ 1 cup stewed tomatoes
- ❖ ½ cup white onion, diced
- ❖ 1/3 cup canola oil
- ❖ 1 teaspoon lemon and pepper seasoning, salt-free
- ❖ 1 teaspoon turmeric

- ❖ 1 teaspoon Mrs. Dash seasoning blend
- ❖ 2 cups of water

Instructions

1. Take a large skillet pan, place it over medium heat, add oil in it and when hot, add garlic and green bell pepper and cook for 4 minutes until sauted.

2. Transfer green pepper mixture to a plate, set aside until needed, then eggplant pieces into the pan and cook for 4 minutes per side until browned, and when done, transfer eggplant to a plate and set aside until needed.

3. Take a medium bowl, place beef in it, add onion, season with all the spices, stir until well combined, and then shape the mixture into 30 small meatballs.

4. Place meatballs into the pan in a single layer and cook for 3 minutes, or until browned.

5. When done, place all the meatballs in the pan, add cooked bell pepper mixture in it along with eggplant, stir in water and tomatoes and simmer for 30 minutes at low heat setting until thoroughly cooked.

6. Serve straight away.

Nutrition Information Per Serving

Calories – 265

Fat – 18 g

Protein – 17 g

Carbohydrates – 12 g

Fiber – 4.6 g

Cholesterol – 47 ml

Net Carbs – 7.4 g

Sodium – 153 mg

Potassium – 598 mg

Phosphorus – 193 mg

Pepper Steak

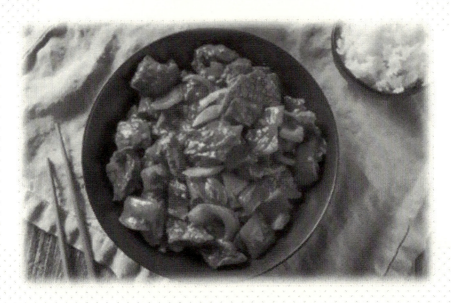

Preparation Time: 10 minutes/Cooking Time: 25minutes/Servings – 6

Ingredients

- ❖ 3 pounds steaks, cut into strips
- ❖ 2 cups green bell pepper, chopped
- ❖ 1 medium white onion, peeled and minced
- ❖ 1 cup carrots, sliced
- ❖ ½ cup celery, chopped
- ❖ 1 package of brown gravy mix
- ❖ 2 tablespoons olive oil
- ❖ 1 ¼ cup water

Instructions

1. Take a large skillet pan, place it over medium-high heat, add oil and when hot, add steak strips and cook for 7 to 10 minutes, or until browned.

2. Then add all the vegetables, pour in ¼ cup water and cook for 8 minutes until softened, covering the pan.

3. Stir in brown gravy mix, then pour in the remaining water, switch the heat to medium heat and cook for 5 minutes until the sauce has reduced to desired thickness.

4. Serve straight away.

Nutrition Information Per Serving

Calories – 340

Fat – 340 g

Protein – 33 g

Carbohydrates – 7 g

Fiber – 2 g

Cholesterol – 81 ml

Net Carbs – 5 g

Sodium – 285 mg

Potassium – 596 mg

Phosphorus – 338 mg

Stuffed Peppers

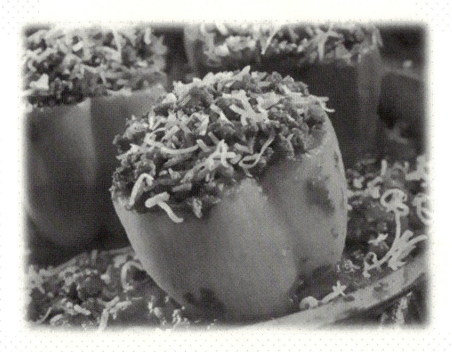

Preparation Time: 10 minutes/Cooking Time: 1 hour and 20 minutes/Servings – 4

Ingredients

- ¾ pound ground beef
- ½ cup white onion, chopped
- 4 medium green bell peppers, destemmed and cored
- 1 tablespoon dried parsley
- 1 ½ teaspoon garlic powder
- 1 teaspoon ground black pepper
- 2 cups cooked white rice
- 3 ounces tomato sauce, unsalted

Instructions

1. Switch on the oven, then set it to 375°F and let it preheat.

2. Take a medium-sized saucepan, place it over medium heat and when hot, add beef and cook for 10 minutes, or until browned.

3. Then drain the excess fat, add remaining ingredients (except for green bell pepper), stir until combined, and simmer for 10 minutes until cooked.

4. When done, spoon the beef mixture evenly between peppers, place the peppers into a baking dish and bake for 1 hour until cooked.

5. Serve straight away.

Nutrition Information Per Serving

Calories – 264

Fat – 7 g

Protein – 20 g

Carbohydrates – 28 g

Fiber – 2.7 g

Cholesterol – 52 ml

Net Carbs – 25.3 g

Sodium – 213 mg

Potassium – 553 mg

Phosphorus – 209 mg

Barley and Beef Stew

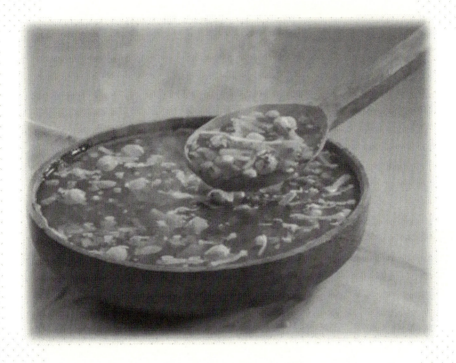

Preparation Time: *10 minutes/****Cooking Time:*** *1 hour and 15 minutes/****Servings*** *– 6*

Ingredients

- ❖ 1 pound beef stew meat, 1 ½ inches, cubed
- ❖ 1 cup pearl barley, soaked for 1 hour
- ❖ ½ cup white onion, diced
- ❖ 2 medium carrots, peeled and sliced
- ❖ 1 large stalk of celery, diced
- ❖ 2 tablespoons all-purpose white flour
- ❖ ½ teaspoon minced garlic
- ❖ ¼ teaspoon ground black pepper

- ❖ ½ teaspoon salt
- ❖ 1 teaspoon onion herb seasoning
- ❖ 2 tablespoons canola oil
- ❖ 2 bay leaves
- ❖ 8 cups of water

Instructions

1. Place beef in a plastic bag, add flour and black pepper, seal the bag and shake well until well coated.

2. Take a large pot, place it over medium heat, add oil and when hot, add coated beef and cook for 10 minutes until browned.

3. When done, transfer beef to a plate, then add celery, onion, and garlic, cook for 2 minutes, pour in water and bring the mixture to a boil.

4. Add beef into boiling mixture, then switch heat to medium level, season with salt, add bay leaf and barley to the pot, stir until mixed and cook for 1 hour until cooked through, stirring every 15 minutes.

5. When done, add carrots, stir in herb seasoning, continue cooking for 1 hour and then serve.

Nutrition Information Per Serving

Calories – 246

Fat – 8 g

Protein – 22 g

Carbohydrates – 21 g

Fiber – 6.3 g

Cholesterol – 51 ml

Net Carbs – 14.7 g

Sodium – 222 mg

Potassium – 369 mg

Phosphorus – 175 mg

Chicken and Corn Soup

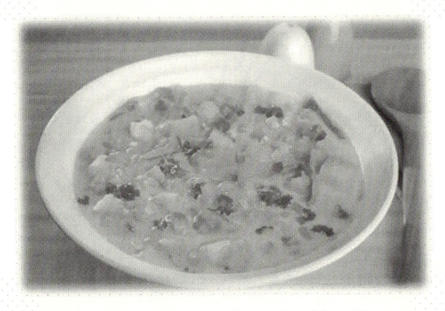

Preparation Time: 15 minutes/Cooking Time: 60 minutes/Servings – 12

Ingredients

* ❖ 6 ounces flat noodles, medium-sized, cooked
* ❖ 4-pound roasting chicken
* ❖ 10 ounces cooked corn
* ❖ ¼ teaspoon ground black pepper
* ❖ 1 tablespoon parsley, chopped
* ❖ 14 cups water

Instructions

1. Take a large pot, place it over medium heat, pour in 8 cups water, add chicken, cook for 30 to 40 minutes until the chicken has cooked, and when done, separate chicken from broth and set aside until needed.

2. Meanwhile, cook the noodles until tender, omit the salt and when cooked, drain the noodles, and set aside until required.

3. Remove fat from the chicken broth by skimming it, let the chicken cool slightly, and then cut it into bite-size pieces.

4. Take a large pot, place it over medium heat, pour in broth and remaining water, stir in chicken, add cooked noodles and corn, stir in black pepper and parsley and simmer for 15 to 20 minutes until hot.

5. When done, ladle soup into bowls and then serve.

Nutrition Information Per Serving

Calories – 222

Fat – 6 g

Protein – 25 g

Carbohydrates – 17 g

Fiber – 1.4 g

Cholesterol – 67 ml

Net Carbs – 15.6 g

Sodium – 240 mg

Potassium – 303 mg

Phosphorus – 212 mg

Asparagus, Chicken and Wild Rice Soup

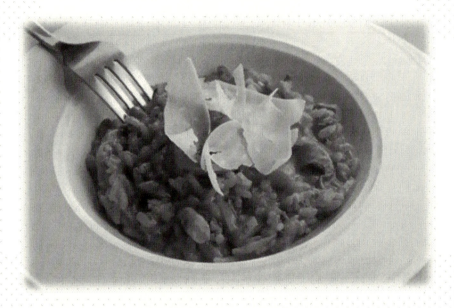

Preparation Time: 10 minutes/Cooking Time: 45 minutes/Servings – 8

Ingredients

- ❖ 2 cups cooked chicken
- ❖ ¾ cup wild rice and white rice blend, cooked
- ❖ ½ cup all-purpose white flour
- ❖ 2 cups asparagus, diced
- ❖ 1 cup carrots, diced
- ❖ ½ cup white onion, diced
- ❖ 1 ½ teaspoon minced garlic
- ❖ ½ teaspoon salt

- ❖ ½ teaspoon dried thyme
- ❖ ½ teaspoon ground black pepper
- ❖ ½ teaspoon ground nutmeg
- ❖ 1 bay leaf
- ❖ ¼ cup unsalted butter
- ❖ ½ cup dry vermouth
- ❖ 4 cups chicken broth, low-sodium
- ❖ 4 cups almond milk, unenriched, unsweetened

Instructions

1. Take a Dutch oven, place it over medium heat, add butter and when it melts, add onion and garlic and cook for 5 minutes, or until tender.
2. Then add carrots, stir in all the spices and herbs and continue cooking for 5 minutes, or until carrots are tender.
3. Switch to low heat, stir in flour, continue cooking for 10 minutes, then pour in vermouth and chicken broth and whisk until combined.
4. Add chicken and asparagus, then gradually stir in milk and continue simmering for 20 minutes until cooked.
5. When done, fold rice into the soup and then serve.

Nutrition Information Per Serving

Calories – 295 *Cholesterol – 45 ml*

Fat – 11 g *Net Carbs – 24.7 g*

Protein – 21 g

Carbohydrates – 28 g

Fiber – 3.3 g

Sodium – 385 mg

Potassium – 527 mg

Phosphorus – 252 mg

Green Chili Stew

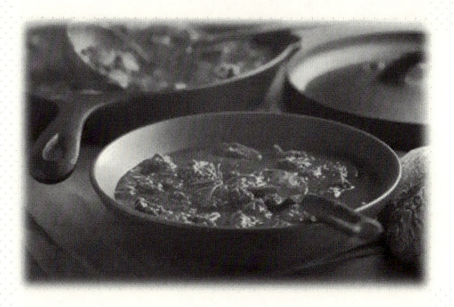

Preparation Time: 10 minutes/Cooking Time: 10 hours and 10 minutes/Servings – 6

Ingredients

- ❖ 1 pound pork chops, cubed
- ❖ 8 ounces green chilies, diced
- ❖ ¾ cup iceberg lettuce, shredded
- ❖ ½ cup all-purpose white flour
- ❖ ¼ cup cilantro, chopped
- ❖ ½ teaspoon minced garlic
- ❖ 1 tablespoon garlic powder
- ❖ 1 teaspoon ground black pepper
- ❖ 1 tablespoon olive oil

- ❖ 6 tablespoons sour cream
- ❖ 14 ounces chicken broth, low-sodium
- ❖ 6 flour tortillas, burrito-size

Instructions

1. Place flour in a large plastic bag, add black pepper and garlic powder, then add pork cubes. Seal the bag and shake well until coated.

2. Take a large skillet pan, place it over medium heat, add oil and when hot, add pork pieces and cook for 10 minutes, or until browned.

3. Switch on the slow cooker, place pork in it, add garlic and chilies, pour in the broth, shut with the lid, and cook pork for 10 hours at low heat setting until tender.

4. When done, place ¾ cup of pork on the tortilla, then roll it like a burrito and serve with lettuce, cilantro, and sour cream.

Nutrition Information Per Serving

Calories – 420

Fat – 16 g

Protein – 25 g

Carbohydrates – 44 g

Fiber – 3.2 g

Cholesterol – 45 ml

Net Carbs – 41.8 g

Sodium – 552 mg

Potassium – 454 mg

Phosphorus – 323 mg

Pumpkin Chili

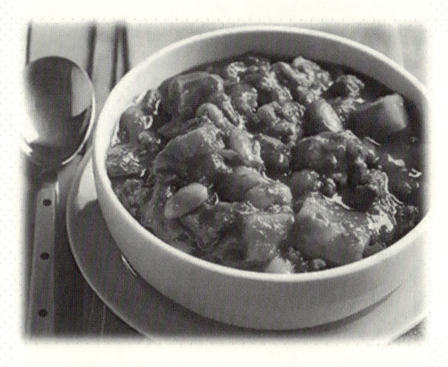

Preparation Time: 10 minutes/Cooking Time: 1 hour and 15 minutes/Servings – 10

Ingredients

- ❖ 2 pounds ground turkey
- ❖ 1 cup cooked kidney beans
- ❖ ½ cup white onion, chopped
- ❖ ½ cup green chilies, chopped
- ❖ ½ cup celery, chopped
- ❖ ½ cup carrot, sliced

- ❖ 1 ½ teaspoon minced garlic
- ❖ 1 tablespoon red chili powder
- ❖ 1 teaspoon dried oregano
- ❖ 2 teaspoons cumin
- ❖ 2 bay leaves
- ❖ 2 tablespoons olive oil
- ❖ 15 ounces pumpkin puree
- ❖ 3 cups chicken broth, low-sodium

Instructions

1. Take a large pot, place it over medium heat, add 1 tablespoon oil in it and when hot, add carrot, celery, onion, and garlic and cook for 5 minutes until tender and when done, transfer vegetables to a plate and set aside until needed.

2. Add remaining oil into the pot, add ground turkey, and cook for 8 minutes, or until meat is no longer pink.

3. Then stir in cooked vegetables along with remaining ingredients, stir until mixed, switch to low heat, and cook for 1 hour, covering the pot.

4. When cooked, remove bay leaf from the chili, then ladle it into bowls and serve.

Nutrition Information Per Serving

Calories – 168

Fat – 5 g

Protein – 24 g

Carbohydrates – 7 g

Fiber – 3.5 g

Cholesterol – 39 ml

Net Carbs – 3.5 g

Sodium – 200 mg

Potassium – 476 mg

Phosphorus – 215 mg

Cauliflower Manchurian

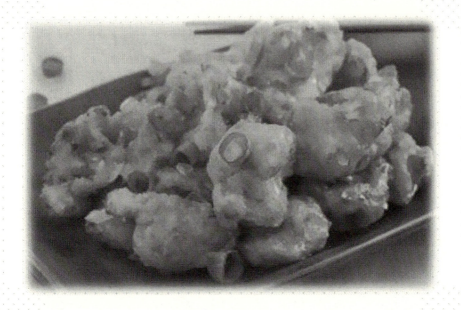

Preparation Time: 10 minutes/Cooking Time: 50 minutes/Servings – 6

Ingredients

> 1 medium head of cauliflower, cut into florets
> 1-inch piece of ginger root, grated
> ½ teaspoon minced garlic
> 1 teaspoon curry powder
> ½ teaspoon red chili powder
> ½ teaspoon cumin powder
> 2 tablespoons rice flour
> 1 teaspoon lemon juice
> 4 cups canola oil

Instructions

1. Take a heatproof bowl, place cauliflower florets in it, and microwave for 12 minutes at medium heat setting until soft.

2. Then add flour, ginger, garlic, and all the spices, and then stir until well coated.

3. Take a deep pan, place it over medium-high heat, add oil and when hot, add coated cauliflower florets in it and cook for 5 minutes, or until golden-brown.

4. When cooked, transfer cauliflower florets to a plate lined with paper towels, cook remaining cauliflower in the same manner and then drizzle with lemon juice.

5. Serve straight away.

Nutrition Information Per Serving

Calories – 77

Fat – 5 g

Protein – 2 g

Carbohydrates – 6 g

Fiber – 1.9 g

Cholesterol – 0 ml

Net Carbs – 4.1 g

Sodium – 23 mg

Potassium – 225 mg

Phosphorus – 36 mg

Eggplant Casserole

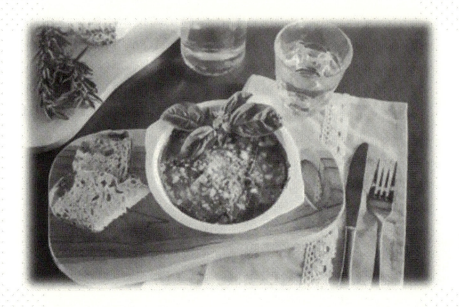

Preparation Time: 10 minutes/Cooking Time: 35 minute/Servings – 4

Ingredients

- ❖ 3 cups eggplant, diced
- ❖ ⅛ teaspoon salt
- ❖ ¼ teaspoon dried sage
- ❖ ½ teaspoon ground black pepper
- ❖ ½ cup breadcrumbs
- ❖ ½ cup liquid creamer, non-dairy
- ❖ 1 tablespoon margarine
- ❖ 3 eggs

Instructions

1. Switch on the oven, then set it to 350°F and let it preheat.

2. Meanwhile, place a large pot half full with water over medium heat, bring it to a boil, then add eggplant pieces, cook for 5 to 8 minutes until boiled, and then drain them.

3. Transfer eggplant pieces to a bowl, mash with a fork, whisk in salt, black pepper, sage, creamer, and eggs until mixed and then spoon the mixture into a greased casserole dish.

4. Place a small frying pan over medium heat, add margarine and when it melts, add breadcrumbs and cook for 3 minutes until golden.

5. Spread breadcrumbs on top of eggplant mixture, then bake for 20 minutes until cooked through, and the top begins to look golden-brown.

6. Serve straight away.

Nutrition Information Per Serving

Calories – 186

Fat – 9 g

Protein – 7 g

Carbohydrates –19 g

Fiber – 1.9 g

Cholesterol – 124 ml

Net Carbs – 17.1 g

Sodium – 246 mg

Potassium – 224 mg

Phosphorus – 115 mg

Pineapple and Pepper Curry

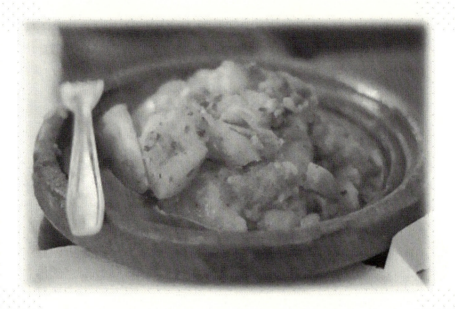

Preparation Time: 5 minutes/Cooking Time: 25 minutes/Servings – 4

Ingredients

- ❖ 5 cherry tomatoes, halved
- ❖ 2 cups green bell pepper, chopped
- ❖ ½ cup pineapple pieces, with juice
- ❖ ½ cup red onion, chopped
- ❖ 1 tablespoon cilantro, chopped
- ❖ 1 tablespoon ginger root, grated
- ❖ 1 teaspoon curry powder
- ❖ ½ tablespoon lemon juice
- ❖ 2 tablespoons olive oil

Instructions

1. Take a medium-sized skillet pan and place it over medium heat, add oil and when hot, add onion and ginger, and cook for 7 minutes, or until softened.

2. Meanwhile, place the peppers in a heatproof bowl and microwave for 6 minutes on a high heat setting.

3. Add peppers into the onion mixture, stir well, switch to low heat, and cook for 10 minutes, stirring frequently.

4. Stir in pineapple pieces, simmer for 2 minutes, then stir in cilantro and curry powder, stir again and simmer for 2 minutes until cooked.

5. When done, drizzle with lemon juice, garnish with cherry tomatoes, and then serve.

Nutrition Information Per Serving

Calories – 107

Fat – 7 g

Protein – 1 g

Carbohydrates – 10 g

Fiber – 1.9 g

Cholesterol – 0 ml

Net Carbs – 8.1 g

Sodium – 4 mg

Potassium – 232 mg

Phosphorus – 26 mg

Ratatouille

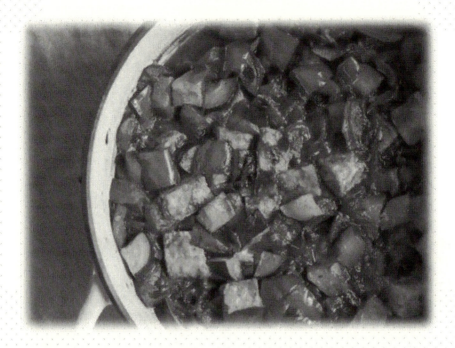

Preparation Time: 10 minutes/Cooking Time: 50 minutes/Servings – 16

Ingredients

- ❖ 3 cups crookneck yellow squash, diced
- ❖ 2 cups white onion, diced
- ❖ 1 medium eggplant, diced
- ❖ 2 cups zucchini squash, diced
- ❖ 1 tablespoon sage leaves
- ❖ 2 medium carrots, peeled and diced
- ❖ 1 tablespoon rosemary leaves
- ❖ 1 medium green bell pepper, cored and diced

- ❖ 1 tablespoon oregano leaves
- ❖ 1 medium yellow bell pepper, cored and diced
- ❖ 1 tablespoon basil leaves
- ❖ 1 medium red bell pepper, cored and diced
- ❖ 2 teaspoons minced garlic
- ❖ 2 tablespoons olive oil
- ❖ 1 cup tomatoes, diced
- ❖ 1 tablespoon ground black pepper
- ❖ 1 tablespoon thyme leaves
- ❖ 8 tablespoons parmesan cheese, grated

Instructions

1. Take a large skillet pan, place it over medium heat, add oil and when hot, add carrots, garlic, and all the herbs, season with black pepper and cook for 2 minutes.
2. Then add remaining vegetables, except for cherry tomatoes, stir and cook for 15 minutes, or until vegetables are tender-crisp.
3. Add tomatoes and cheese, stir until well mixed and simmer for 30 minutes until thoroughly cooked, covering the pan.
4. Serve straight away.

Nutrition Information Per Serving

Calories – 54

Fat – 3 g

Protein – 3 g

Carbohydrates – 6 g

Fiber – 2.4 g

Cholesterol – 2 ml

Net Carbs – 3.6 g

Sodium – 84 mg

Potassium – 302 mg

Phosphorus – 58 mg

Brussels Sprouts with Pears

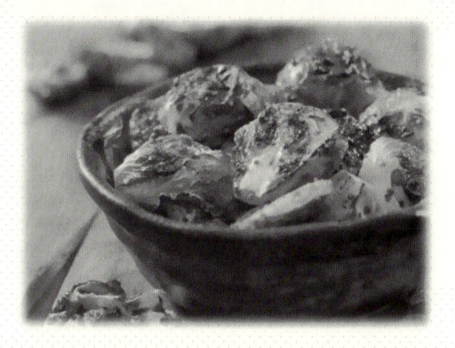

Preparation Time: 10 minutes/Cooking Time: 24 minutes/Servings – 4

Ingredients

- ❖ 2 ½ cups Brussel sprouts, halved
- ❖ 2 medium pears, ½-inch cubed, peeled
- ❖ 2 teaspoons olive oil
- ❖ 1 teaspoon balsamic vinegar glaze

Instructions

1. Switch on the oven, then set it to 400°F, and let it preheat.

2. Take a large bowl, add 1 teaspoon oil to it, then add sprouts and toss until well coated.

3. Take a 9 by 13 inches sheet pan, spread sprouts on one half in a single layer, and then bake for 12 minutes.

4. Add remaining oil in the bowl, add pear pieces to it, toss until well coated, and after 12 minutes, place pears on the empty side of the sheet pan and continue roasting for another 12 minutes, or until vegetables are tender.

5. When done, drizzle glaze over the pears, toss them with sprouts, and then serve.

Nutrition Information Per Serving

Calories – 110

Fat – 3 g

Protein – 2 g

Carbohydrates – 19 g

Fiber – 100 g

Cholesterol – 0ml

Net Carbs – 17 g

Sodium – 15 mg

Potassium – 320 mg

Phosphorus – 49 mg

Stuffed Zucchini

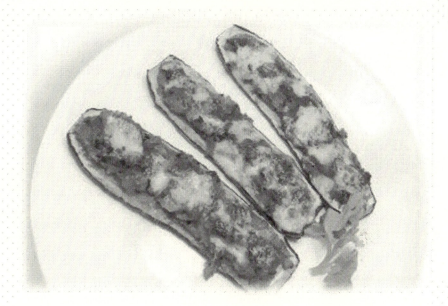

Preparation Time: 10 minutes/Cooking Time: 28

minutes/Servings – 2

Ingredients

- ❖ 4 slices of white bread, toasted
- ❖ 2 medium zucchini
- ❖ ¼ teaspoon dried sage
- ❖ 1 teaspoon onion powder
- ❖ 1 teaspoon dill weed
- ❖ 1 teaspoon lemon and pepper seasoning, salt-free
- ❖ 1 teaspoon Dash seasoning blend

Instructions

1. Prepare the zucchini by cutting each into half, lengthwise, and then scooping out the seeds to create a trench.

2. Take a medium-sized pot half full with water, place it over medium heat, bring it to a boil, then add zucchini in it and boil for 3 to 5 minutes.

3. Meanwhile, toast the bread slices, then transfer it to a food processor and pulse until the mixture resembles crumbs.

4. Transfer breadcrumbs in a bowl, add sage, onion powder, dill, lemon and pepper, and Dash seasoning, and stir until mixed.

5. Drain the zucchini, pour ½ cup of the cooking liquid into the breadcrumbs mixture and blend with a fork until combined.

6. Take an 8-by-8 inches baking dish, place zucchini halves in it, peel side down, spoon breadcrumbs mixture into the zucchini, and then bake for 20 minutes until cooked.

7. Serve straight away.

Nutrition Information Per Serving

Calories – 82

Fat – 1 g

Protein – 3 g

Carbohydrates – 15 g

Fiber – 1.7 g

Cholesterol – 0 ml

Net Carbs – 13.3 g

Sodium – 180 mg

Potassium – 276 mg

Phosphorus – 63 mg

Thai Red Curry Vegetables and Rice

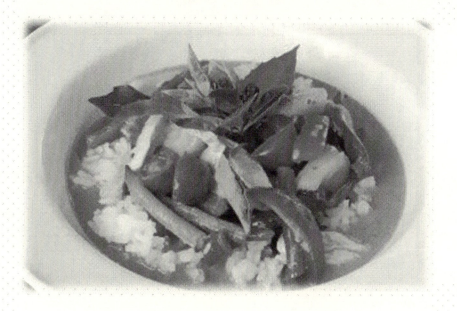

Preparation Time: 10 minutes/Cooking Time: 50 minutes/Servings – 4

Ingredients

- ❖ 2 cups cooked white rice
- ❖ 1 cup green beans, diced
- ❖ 1 small shallot, peeled and minced
- ❖ 2 cups cauliflower florets
- ❖ 2 medium carrots, sliced
- ❖ 1 lime, cut into wedges
- ❖ 1 lime leaf, dried
- ❖ 2 tablespoons Thai red curry paste

- ❖ 1 tablespoon canola oil

- ❖ 14 ounces vegetable broth, low-sodium

- ❖ 8 ounces coconut milk, unsweetened

Instructions

1. Take a large pot, place it over low heat, add oil and when hot, add shallots and cook for 8 minutes, or until tender.

2. Then stir in red curry paste, continue cooking for 1 minute until fragrant, add a lime leaf, pour in broth and milk, stir until mixed, and bring the mixture to a boil.

3. Add all the vegetables, stir until mixed, simmer for 12 minutes until vegetables are fork-tender and when done, remove the pot from the heat and remove the lime leaf.

4. Distribute rice between bowls, top with cooked vegetables and the sauce, and serve with lime wedges.

Nutrition Information Per Serving

Calories – 210

Fat – 17 g

Protein – 8 g

Carbohydrates – 26 g

Fiber – 4.8 g

Cholesterol – 0 ml

Net Carbs – 20.2 g

Sodium – 277 mg

Potassium – 588 mg

Phosphorus – 142 mg

Vegetable Paella

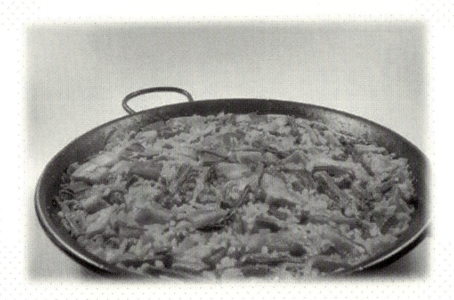

Preparation Time: 5minutes/Cooking Time: 20 minutes/Servings – 8

Ingredients

- ❖ 4 cups cooked white rice
- ❖ 2 cups asparagus
- ❖ ½ cup white onion, chopped
- ❖ 1 cup green bell pepper, chopped
- ❖ 3 cups broccoli florets
- ❖ 1 ½ cup zucchini, chopped
- ❖ ½ teaspoon salt
- ❖ 1 tablespoon olive oil
- ❖ ½ teaspoon saffron

Instructions

1. Take a large pot, add broccoli and asparagus, pour in water to cover the vegetables, boil them for 4 minutes until tender-crisp, and then drain them.

2. Take a large skillet pan, place it over medium heat, add oil and when hot, add boiled vegetables along with onion, zucchini, and bell pepper and cook for 5 minutes until tender-crisp.

3. Then add remaining ingredients, stir until mixed and continue cooking for 5 minutes until hot.

4. Serve straight away.

Nutrition Information Per Serving

Calories – 146

Fat – 2 g

Protein – 5 g

Carbohydrates – 26 g

Fiber – 1.8 g

Cholesterol – 0 ml

Net Carbs – 24.2 g

Sodium – 150 mg

Potassium – 305 mg

Phosphorus – 89 mg

Rice-Stuffed Chicken

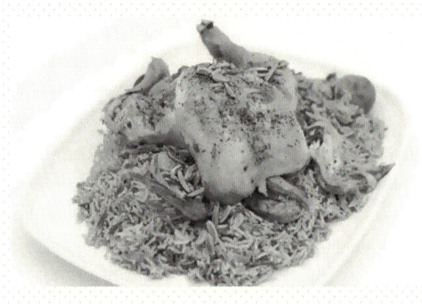

Preparation Time: 10 minutes/Cooking Time: 1 hour and 30 minutes/Servings – 6

Ingredients

- ❖ 4 pounds whole chicken, cleaned
- ❖ 2 scallions, chopped
- ❖ ½ cup green bell pepper, chopped
- ❖ 1 cup pineapple pieces
- ❖ ⅔ cup white rice
- ❖ 1 teaspoon ground black pepper
- ❖ 1 tablespoon Worcestershire sauce
- ❖ 1 tablespoon olive oil
- ❖ ¼ cup pineapple juice

Instructions

1. Switch on the oven, then set it to 350°F and let it preheat.

2. Meanwhile, clean the whole chicken, pat dry with paper towels, and then brush well with oil.

3. Place the rice in a bowl, add scallions, bell pepper, pineapple, black pepper, oil, and Worcestershire sauce, stir until mixed, and then spoon this mixture into the cavity of the chicken.

4. Take a roasting pan, place stuffed chicken in it and bake for 1 hour and 30 minutes until the internal temperature of the chicken reaches 180° and the temperature of the rice stuffing reach 165°.

5. When done, let roasted chicken rest for 15 minutes, then spoon the rice stuffing to a serving dish, cut chicken into pieces, and serve.

Nutrition Information Per Serving

Calories – 323	Cholesterol – 86 ml
Fat – 17 g	Net Carbs – 23.2 g
Protein – 28 g	Sodium – 118 mg
Carbohydrates – 24 g	Potassium – 344 mg
Fiber – 0.8 g	Phosphorus – 220 mg

Apple and Chicken Curry

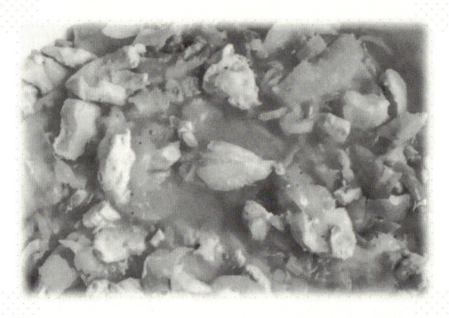

Preparation Time: 15 minutes/Cooking Time: 1 hour and 10 minutes/Servings – 8

Ingredients

- ❖ 1 medium apple: peeled, cored, chopped
- ❖ 8 skinless chicken breast
- ❖ 1 small white onion, peeled and chopped
- ❖ ½ teaspoon minced garlic
- ❖ 3 tablespoons all-purpose white flour
- ❖ ½ tablespoon dried basil
- ❖ ¼ teaspoon ground black pepper
- ❖ 1 tablespoon curry powder
- ❖ 3 tablespoons unsalted butter

- ❖ 1 cup chicken broth, low-sodium
- ❖ 1 cup rice milk, unenriched

Instructions

1. Switch on the oven, then set it to 350°F and let it preheat.
2. Take a 9-by-13 inch baking dish, grease it with oil, place chicken in it in a single layer. Sprinkle with black pepper and set aside until required.
3. Take a medium-sized saucepan, place it over medium heat, add butter and when it melts, add onion and apple and cook for 5 minutes, or until tender.
4. Season with basil and curry powder, cook for 1 minute until saute, and then stir in flour, continue cooking for 1 minute.
5. Pour in milk and broth, stir until combined, remove the pan from heat, pour this sauce over chicken, and then bake for 60 minutes until thoroughly cooked.
6. Serve straight away.

Nutrition Information Per Serving

Calories – 232

Cholesterol – 85 ml

Fat – 8 g

Net Carbs – 9.8 g

Protein – 29 g

Sodium – 118 mg

Carbohydrates – 11 g

Potassium – 323 mg

Fiber – 1.2 g

Phosphorus – 225 mg

Chicken with Garlic Sauce

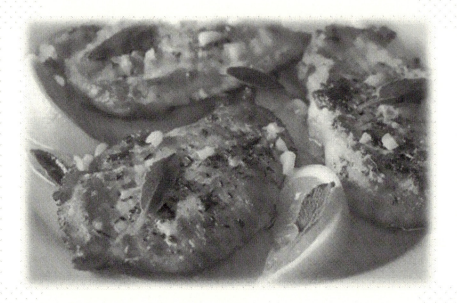

Preparation Time: 10 minutes/Cooking Time: 30 minutes/Servings – 8

Ingredients

- ❖ 8 skinless chicken breasts
- ❖ 1 medium head of garlic, peeled and sliced
- ❖ ½ teaspoon ground black pepper
- ❖ 1 tablespoon rosemary leaves, chopped
- ❖ ½ cup balsamic vinegar
- ❖ 2 tablespoons olive oil
- ❖ ½ cup white wine
- ❖ 2 cups chicken broth, low-sodium

Instructions

1. Take a 9-by-13 inches baking dish, add rosemary, wine, and vinegar, pour in the broth, stir until mixed, add chicken, toss it well and let it marinate for a minimum of 4 hours.

2. Then take a large saute pan, place it over medium-high heat, add oil and when hot, add sliced garlic and cook for 4 minutes, or until golden.

3. Transfer garlic to a plate, set aside until needed, switch to high heat, add marinated chicken in it, sprinkle with black pepper, and cook for 1 minute per side until golden.

4. Then switch to medium heat, pour marinade over the chicken, add garlic and simmer the chicken for 15 minutes until cooked, turning halfway.

5. When done, transfer chicken to a dish, switch to high heat, and bring the sauce to a boil, then switch heat to medium-high and simmer the liquid until thickened.

6. Drizzle liquid over chicken and then serve.

Nutrition Information Per Serving

Calories – 210	Cholesterol – 70 ml
Fat – 7 g	Net Carbs – 3.8 g
Protein – 28 g	Sodium – 85 mg
Carbohydrates – 4 g	Potassium – 277 mg
Fiber – 0.2 g	Phosphorus – 208 mg

Chicken Pot Pie

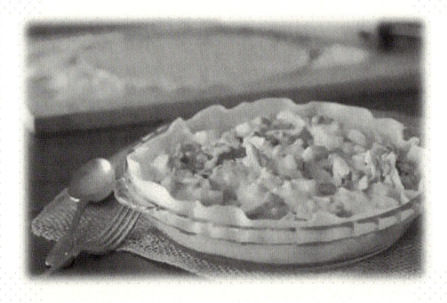

Preparation Time: 10 minutes/Cooking Time: 1 hour and 15 minutes/Servings – 8

Ingredients

- ❖ 12-ounce farfalle pasta
- ❖ 1 ½ cup carrots, sliced
- ❖ 2 pounds skinless chicken breasts
- ❖ 1 cup celery, diced
- ❖ 2 cups potatoes, diced
- ❖ 1 cup white onion, diced
- ❖ 12 cups water
- ❖ ¼ teaspoon ground black pepper
- ❖ ½ teaspoon dried thyme
- ❖ 2 tablespoons parsley, chopped

Instructions

1. Take a large saucepan, place it over medium-high heat, add chicken, stir in all the seasoning, pour in water, bring it to a boil, then switch to medium-low heat and simmer for 45 minutes.

2. Meanwhile, take a large pot, place it over medium-high heat, place potatoes in it, pour in water to cover the potatoes, and bring it to a boil.

3. Then drain the water, cover potatoes with fresh water, bring it to a boil, and continue cooking for 10 minutes. When done, drain the potatoes and set aside until required.

4. When the chicken has cooked, remove the pan from heat, then remove chicken from it and set aside until required.

5. Remove fat from the broth by skimming it, then place the pan over medium-high heat, add carrot, onion, and celery, bring it to a boil, and then cook for 5 minutes.

6. Add potatoes and pasta, stir in parsley, and boil for 14 minutes, or until pasta is tender.

7. Cut the chicken into bite-sized pieces, add into the pan, stir and cook until thoroughly heated.

8. Serve straight away.

Nutrition Information Per Serving

Calories – 335

Fat – 4 g

Protein – 32 g

Carbohydrates – 42 g

Fiber – 3.3 g

Cholesterol – 70 ml

Net Carbs – 38.7 g

Sodium – 118 mg

Potassium – 521 mg

Phosphorus – 290 mg

Chicken with Mushroom Sauce

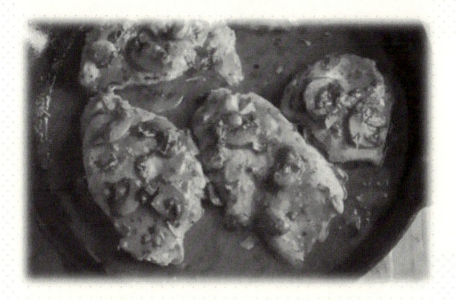

Preparation Time: 10 minutes/Cooking Time: 55 minutes/Servings – 4

Ingredients

- 1 ¼ pound skinless chicken breast
- 1 cup mushrooms, sliced
- 2 bulbs of garlic
- ½ teaspoon salt
- ½ teaspoon dried thyme
- ¼ teaspoon ground black pepper
- ½ cup all-purpose white flour
- ¼ cup butter, unsalted
- 2 teaspoons olive oil

- ½ cup whole milk, unsweetened
- 1 ½ cups chicken broth, low-sodium

Instructions

1. Switch on the oven, then set it to 350°F and let it preheat.

2. Cut the top from each bulb of garlic, place bulb on a large piece of foil, cut-side up, drizzle with oil, wrap bulbs tightly, and then bake for 45 minutes, or until tender.

3. Meanwhile, wrap each chicken breast in a plastic wrap, and then pound with a meat mallet until ¼-inch thick.

4. Place flour in a shallow dish, stir in salt, thyme, and black pepper until combined, reserve 3 tablespoons of this mixture, and use the remaining mixture to coat the chicken.

5. Then take a large skillet pan, place it over medium-high heat, add 2 tablespoons butter and when it melts, add chicken and cook for 8 minutes until internal temperature of the chicken reaches 165°F, flipping halfway, and when done, transfer chicken to a plate, cover with foil to keep it warm, and set aside until needed.

6. When the garlic has baked, cool garlic bulbs for 10 minutes, then gently squeeze the cloves, chop the garlic, and set aside until required.

7. Add remaining butter in a skillet pan and when it melts, add mushrooms and cook for 5 minutes, or until golden-brown.

8. Sprinkle the reserved flour mixture over mushrooms, stir, cook for 2 minutes, add garlic, pour in milk and broth, stir until well combined, and bring the mixture to a boil.

9. Switch to low heat, simmer mushroom sauce for 3 minutes until sauce has thickened slightly, add chicken, toss until well coated with the sauce, and cook for 2 minutes until hot.

10. Serve straight away.

Nutrition Information Per Serving

Calories – 388

Fat – 19 g

Protein – 35 g

Carbohydrates – 20 g

Fiber – 1 g

Cholesterol – 112 ml

Net Carbs – 19 g

Sodium – 259 mg

Potassium – 486 mg

Phosphorus – 319 mg

Chicken in Herb Sauce

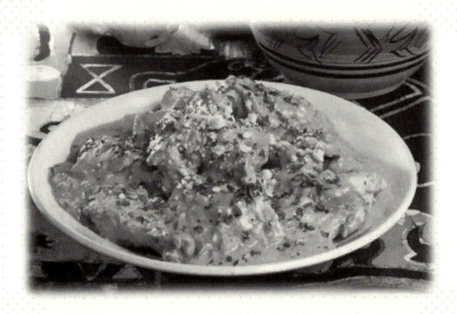

Preparation Time: 10 minutes/Cooking Time: 33 minutes/Servings – 2

Ingredients

- ❖ 2 skinless chicken breasts
- ❖ ½ teaspoon garlic powder
- ❖ ¼ teaspoon celery salt
- ❖ ¼ teaspoon ground black pepper
- ❖ ½ teaspoon paprika
- ❖ ¼ teaspoon celery seeds
- ❖ ½ teaspoon mustard powder
- ❖ 3 tablespoons lemon juice
- ❖ 2 tablespoons butter, unsalted
- ❖ 1 tablespoon parmesan cheese, grated

Instructions

1. Switch on the oven, then set it to 350°F and let it preheat.

2. Meanwhile, take a small saucepan, place it over medium heat, add butter and when it melts, add all the ingredients (except for chicken and cheese), stir until mixed, and cook the sauce for 1 minute until hot.

3. Remove pan from heat, and then stir in cheese until it melts.

4. Take a baking dish, place chicken breasts in it, cover with prepared sauce, turn the chicken to coat it in the sauce, and then bake for 30 minutes until chicken is thoroughly cooked.

5. Serve straight away.

Nutrition Information Per Serving

Calories – 272

Fat – 16 g

Protein – 28 g

Carbohydrates – 3 g

Fiber – 0.5 g

Cholesterol – 107 ml

Net Carbs – 2.5 g

Sodium – 292 mg

Potassium – 284 mg

Phosphorus – 228 mg

Drinks

Hot Cocoa

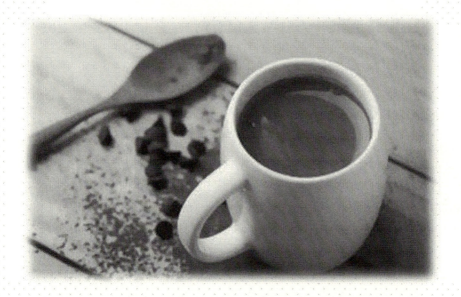

Preparation Time: 10 minutes/Cooking Time: 5 minutes/Servings – 1

Ingredients

- ❖ 1 tablespoon cocoa powder, unsweetened
- ❖ 2 teaspoons Splenda granulated sugar
- ❖ 3 tablespoons whipped dessert topping
- ❖ 1 cup water, at room temperature
- ❖ 2 tablespoons water, cold

Instructions

1. Take a saucepan, place it over medium heat, and let it heat until hot.
2. Take a cup, place cocoa powder and sugar in it, pour in cold water, and mix well.
3. Then slowly stir in hot water until cocoa mixture dissolves and top with whipped topping.
4. Serve straight away.

Nutrition Information Per Serving

Calories – 72

Fat – 3 g

Protein – 1 g

Carbohydrates – 13 g

Fiber – 1.8 g

Cholesterol – 0 ml

Net Carbs – 11.2 g

Sodium – 10 mg

Potassium – 100 mg

Phosphorus – 49 mg

Rice Milk

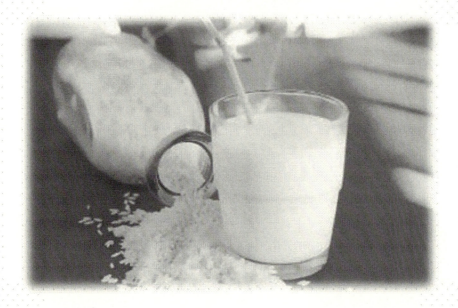

Preparation Time: 5 minutes/Cooking Time: 0 minutes/Servings – 2

Ingredients

- ❖ 1 cup rice milk, unenriched, chilled
- ❖ 1 scoop of vanilla whey protein

Instructions

1. Pour milk in a blender, add whey protein, and then pulse until well blended.
2. Distribute the milk into two glasses and serve.

Nutrition Information Per Serving

Calories – 130

Fat – 2 g

Protein – 14 g

Carbohydrates – 18 g

Fiber – 0 g

Cholesterol – 40 ml

Net Carbs – 18 g

Sodium – 120 mg

Potassium – 127 mg

Phosphorus – 80 mg

Cinnamon and Hazelnut Coffee

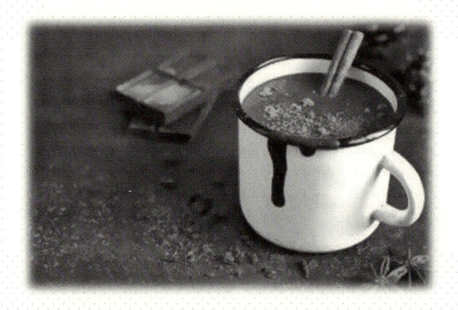

Preparation Time: 0 minutes/Cooking Time: 5 minutes/Servings – 4

Ingredients

- ❖ 4 sticks of cinnamon
- ❖ 8 teaspoons hazelnut syrup, sugar-free
- ❖ 4 tablespoons milk, low-fat
- ❖ 4 cups brewed coffee

Instructions

1. Distribute brewed coffee into small cups, and then stir in 2 teaspoons of hazelnut syrup into each cup along with 1 tablespoon milk until combined.

2. Garnish coffee with a stick of cinnamon and serve.

Nutrition Information Per Serving

Calories – 13

Fat – 0 g

Protein – 1 g

Carbohydrates – 1 g

Fiber – 0 g

Cholesterol – 1 ml

Net Carbs – 1 g

Sodium – 13 mg

Potassium – 139 mg

Phosphorus – 22 mg

Almond Milk

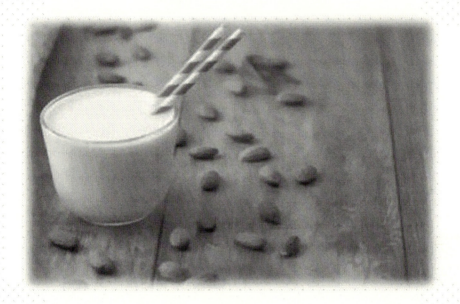

Preparation Time: 5 minutes/Cooking Time: 0 minutes/Servings – 3

Ingredients

- ❖ 1 cup almonds, soaked in warm water for 10 minutes
- ❖ 1 teaspoon vanilla extract, unsweetened
- ❖ 3 cups of filtered water

Instructions

1. Drain the soaked almonds, place them into the blender, pour in water, and blend for 2 minutes until almonds are chopped.

2. Strain the milk by passing it through a cheesecloth into a bowl, discard almond meal, and then stir vanilla into the milk.

3. Cover the milk, refrigerate until chilled, and when ready to serve, stir it well, pour the milk evenly into the glasses and then serve.

Nutrition Information Per Serving

Calories – 40

Fat – 3 g

Protein – 1 g

Carbohydrates – 2 g

Fiber – 0 g

Cholesterol – 0 ml

Net Carbs – 2 g

Sodium – 6 mg

Potassium – 180 mg

Phosphorus – 40 mg

Blueberry Smoothie

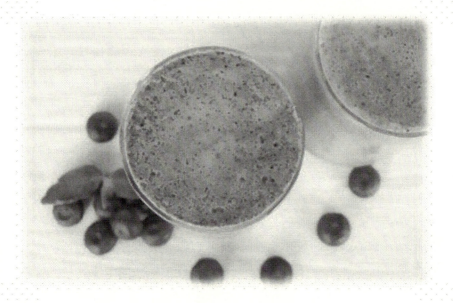

Preparation Time: 5 minutes/Cooking Time: 0 minutes/Servings – 4

Ingredients

- ❖ 1 cup frozen blueberries
- ❖ 6 tablespoons protein powder
- ❖ 8 packets of Splenda
- ❖ 14 ounces of apple juice, unsweetened
- ❖ 8 cubes of ice

Instructions

1. Take a blender, place all the ingredients (in order) in it, and then process for 1 minute until smooth.
2. Distribute the smoothie between four glasses and then serve.

Nutrition Information Per Serving

Calories – 108

Fat – 0 g

Protein – 9 g

Carbohydrates – 18 g

Fiber – 1.2 g

Cholesterol – 0 ml

Net Carbs – 16.8 g

Sodium – 27 mg

Potassium – 183 mg

Phosphorus – 42 mg

Citrus Shake

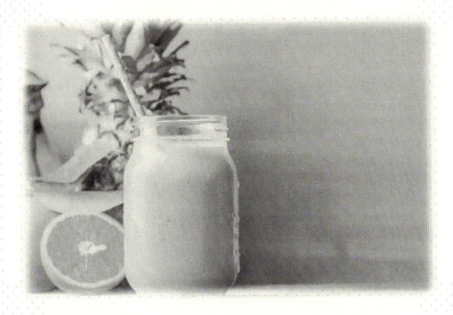

Preparation Time: 10 minutes/Cooking Time: 50 minutes/Servings – 2

Ingredients

- ❖ ½ cup pineapple juice
- ❖ ½ cup almond milk, unsweetened
- ❖ 1 cup orange sherbet
- ❖ ½ cup liquid egg substitute, low-cholesterol

Instructions

1. Take a blender, place all the ingredients (in order) in it, and then process for 30 seconds until smooth.
2. Distribute the shake between two glasses and then serve.

Nutrition Information Per Serving

Calories – 190

Fat – 2 g

Protein – 7 g

Carbohydrates – 36 g

Fiber – 1.3 g

Cholesterol – 1 ml

Net Carbs – 24.7 g

Sodium – 192 mg

Potassium – 310 mg

Phosphorus – 83 mg

Cucumber and Lemon-Flavored Water

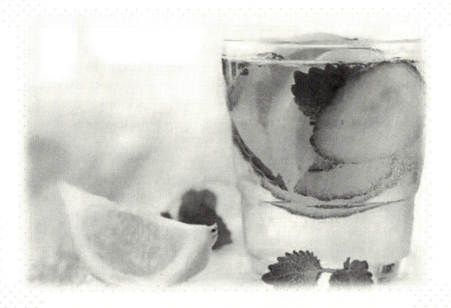

Preparation Time: 3 hours and 5 minutes/Cooking Time:
0 minutes/Servings – 10

Ingredients

- ❖ 1 lemon, deseeded, sliced
- ❖ ¼ cup fresh mint leaves, chopped
- ❖ 1 medium cucumber, sliced
- ❖ ¼ cup fresh basil leaves, chopped
- ❖ 10 cups water

Instructions

1. Take a pitcher, place all the ingredients (in order) in it, and then stir until mixed.
2. Place the pitcher in the refrigerator, chill the water for a minimum of 3 hours (or overnight), and then serve.

Nutrition Information Per Serving

Calories – 4

Fat – 0 g

Protein – 0 g

Carbohydrates – 1 g

Fiber – 0.4 g

Cholesterol – 0 ml

Net Carbs – 0.6 g

Sodium – 8 mg

Potassium – 38 mg

Phosphorus – 4 mg

Fruity Smoothie

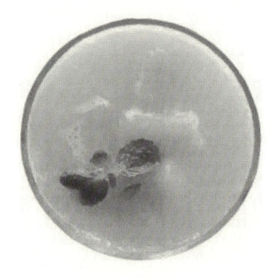

Preparation Time: 10 minutes/Cooking Time: 0

minutes/Servings – 2

Ingredients

❖ 2 scoops vanilla-flavored whey protein powder

❖ 8 ounces fruit cocktail, with juice

❖ 1 cup of water, cold

❖ 1 cup crushed ice

Instructions

1. Take a blender, place all the ingredients (in order) in it, and then process for 30 seconds until smooth.

2. Distribute the shake between two glasses and then serve.

Nutrition Information Per Serving

Calories – 186

Fat – 2 g

Protein – 23 g

Carbohydrates – 19 g

Fiber – 1.1 g

Cholesterol – 41 ml

Net Carbs – 17.9 g

Sodium – 62 mg

Potassium – 282 mg

Phosphorus – 118 mg

Hot Mulled Punch

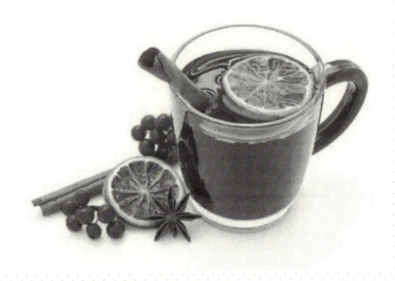

Preparation Time: 5 minutes/Cooking Time: 10 minutes/Servings – 14

Ingredients

- ❖ 4 sticks of cinnamon, broken
- ❖ ½ cup brown sugar
- ❖ 1 ½ teaspoons whole cloves
- ❖ 6 cups cranberry juice, unsweetened
- ❖ 8 cups apple juice, unsweetened

Instructions

1. Take a large pot, place it over medium-high heat, add all the ingredients in it, and stir until mixed.

2. Simmer the punch until hot and then serve.

Nutrition Information Per Serving

Calories – 135

Fat – 0 g

Protein – 0 g

Carbohydrates – 33 g

Fiber – 0.3 g

Cholesterol – 0 ml

Net Carbs – 32.7 g

Sodium – 7 mg

Potassium – 267 mg

Phosphorus – 25 mg

Lemon Smoothie

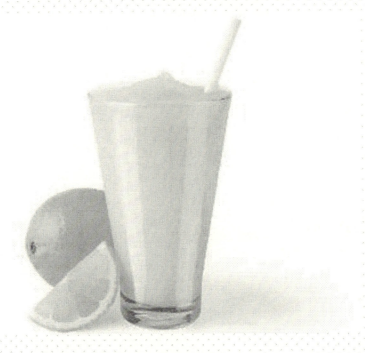

Preparation Time: 5 minutes/Cooking Time: 0 minutes

Servings – 1/

Ingredients

- ❖ 4 teaspoons Splenda granulated sugar
- ❖ 3 tablespoons whipped dessert topping
- ❖ 2 teaspoons lemon juice
- ❖ 8 ounces liquid egg white, pasteurized

Instructions

1. Take a smoothie glass, place all the ingredients in it, and stir well until whipped topping melts.

2. Serve straight away.

Nutrition Information Per Serving

Calories – 227

Fat – 3 g

Protein – 28 g

Carbohydrates – 22 g

Fiber – 0 g

Cholesterol – 0 ml

Net Carbs – 22 g

Sodium – 428 mg

Potassium – 433 mg

Phosphorus – 39 mg

Peach Smoothie

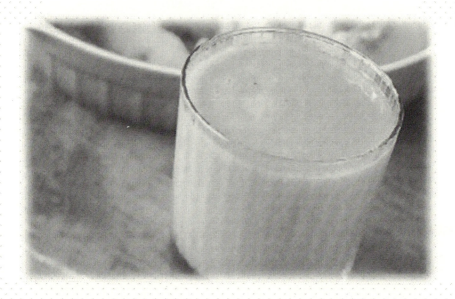

Preparation Time: 5 minutes/Cooking Time: 0 minutes/Servings – 1

Ingredients

- ❖ ¾ cup fresh peaches, diced
- ❖ 1 tablespoon Splenda granulated sugar
- ❖ 2 tablespoons powdered egg whites
- ❖ ½ cup ice

Instructions

1. Take a blender, place peaches in it, and blend for 30 seconds until smooth.

2. Then add remaining ingredients in a blender, pulse for 1 minute until combined, and then pour the smoothie in a glass.

3. Serve straight away.

Nutrition Information Per Serving

Calories – 132

Fat – 0 g

Protein – 10 g

Carbohydrates – 24 g

Fiber – 1.9 g

Cholesterol – 0 ml

Net Carbs – 22.1 g

Sodium – 154 mg

Potassium – 353 mg

Phosphorus – 36 mg

Pineapple Punch

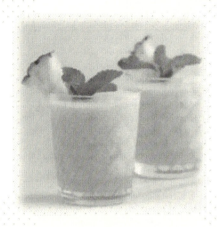

Preparation Time: 5 minutes

Cooking Time: 0 minutes

Servings – 12

Ingredients

- ❖ Pineapple slices as needed for garnishing
- ❖ 8 ounces crushed pineapple
- ❖ 4 cups pineapple juice
- ❖ 4 cups lemon-lime soda
- ❖ 4 cups of ice cubes

Instructions

1. Take a large punch bowl, place all the ingredients in it, and stir until mixed.
2. Pour punch into glasses, add a slice of pineapple, and then serve.

Nutrition Information Per Serving

Calories – 120

Fat – 0 g

Protein – 0 g

Carbohydrates – 30 g

Fiber – 0.1 g

Cholesterol – 0 ml

Net Carbs – 29.9 g

Sodium – 26 mg

Potassium – 106 mg

Phosphorus – 6 mg

Conclusion

People from all over the globe suffer from some kind of disease, but we all have to still keep on living even though it might be a little more difficult. Those who have renal disease can replenish vitamins and necessary nutrients by following a diet. People with mild complications may tweak their food a little bit, however, those with end-stage renal disease must follow a strict diet provided by their doctor.

Even with a disease that limits so many foods, you can still make delicious treats and meals by the alternatives provided. You can also customize them according to your palate so that the food you eat not only helps your body but also boosts your mood. You can share these tasty renal-friendly meals with your friends and family, and live a long life with them by your side!

Made in the USA
Middletown, DE
10 September 2020